ADVANCE PRAISE

"A great combination of fascinating science, simple and effective ways to train the mind, and practical suggestions for daily life. Full of brilliant insights, and always clear, friendly, and encouraging: a real path to greater well-being in a challenging world."

—**Rick Hanson, PhD,** author of *Buddha's Brain*, *Resilient*, and *Hardwiring Happiness*

"It's fitting that this book on happiness is a sheer delight! It will take you through simple exercises that will improve your baseline happiness. You'll feel awe, gratitude, compassion, connection, and peace. Take it seriously, and it will change your life."

—**Marisa G. Franco, PhD,** TED speaker and *NYT*-bestselling author of *Platonic: How the Science of Attachment Can Help You Make—and Keep—Friends*

The Science of Happiness
Workbook

The Science of Happiness
Workbook

Greater Good Science Center

Kira M. Newman

Jill Suttie

Shuka Kalantari

Norton Professional Books

An Imprint of W. W. Norton & Company
Independent Publishers Since 1923

Important Note: *The Science of Happiness Workbook* is intended to provide general information on the subject of health and well-being; it is not a substitute for medical or psychological treatment and may not be relied upon for purposes of diagnosing or treating any illness. Please seek out the care of a professional healthcare provider if you are pregnant, nursing, or experiencing symptoms of any potentially serious condition. As of press time, the URLs displayed in this book link or refer to existing sites. The publisher and author are not responsible for any content that appears on third-party websites.

Copyright © 2025 by The Regents of the University of California

All rights reserved
Printed in the United States of America
First Edition

For information about permission to reproduce selections from this book, write to Permissions, W. W. Norton & Company, Inc., 500 Fifth Avenue, New York, NY 10110

For information about special discounts for bulk purchases, please contact W. W. Norton Special Sales at specialsales@wwnorton.com or 800-233-4830

Manufacturing by Versa Press
Production manager: Gwen Cullen

ISBN: 978-1-324-01920-6

W. W. Norton & Company, Inc., 500 Fifth Avenue, New York, NY 10110
www.wwnorton.com

W. W. Norton & Company Ltd., 15 Carlisle Street, London W1D 3BS

1 2 3 4 5 6 7 8 9 0

To Dad, I wish you could have read this book.
—Kira M. Newman

For my sons, Michael and David, and my husband, Don. You make my life happy, meaningful, and interesting all at once.
—Jill Suttie

To my sons, Sina and Aban, and their baba—thank you for showing me what it is to live a meaningful life.
—Shuka Kalantari

CONTENTS

Acknowledgments   *xi*
Introduction   *xiii*

CHAPTER 1 • Connection   1

CHAPTER 2 • Kindness   18

CHAPTER 3 • Empathy   34

CHAPTER 4 • Compassion   49

CHAPTER 5 • Awe   64

CHAPTER 6 • Mindfulness   80

CHAPTER 7 • Gratitude   96

CHAPTER 8 • Self-Compassion   111

CHAPTER 9 • Emotion Regulation   125

CHAPTER 10 • Purpose   140

Conclusion   *157*
References   *165*
Index   *199*

● ACKNOWLEDGMENTS

This book would not have been possible without the generosity, dedication, and wisdom of so many people.

First, we want to express our deepest gratitude to the researchers whose work forms the foundation of this book and the practices we include. Their dedication to studying the science of human flourishing has provided invaluable insights into what it means to live well, and we are honored to share their findings.

We are grateful to the guests of *The Science of Happiness* podcast and the students of The Science of Happiness course who have shared their personal experiences with these practices. Their stories bring the research to life and help us better understand what it looks like to pursue a meaningful life and a compassionate society.

We also extend our heartfelt appreciation to the team at Norton for their support in bringing this book into the world, starting with an idea many years ago.

To our current and former colleagues at the Greater Good Science Center, thank you for your commitment to making the science of a meaningful life accessible and actionable, and for always being there for us with your thoughtfulness, support, and humor. We love our GGSC family!

We are especially grateful to Emiliana Simon-Thomas, the coinstructor of The Science of Happiness course for more than a decade, who originally brought us the idea for this workbook and lent her scientific expertise along the way; to her coinstructor Dacher Keltner and *The Science of Happiness* podcast team; and to Jason Marsh, who helped shape the initial vision for the book. A special thanks to Hannah Villareal for gathering research on the practices and offering thoughtful feedback on several chapters.

And, of course, to our families—thank you for your patience, encouragement, and love as we worked to bring this book to life.

To all those who contributed—whether through research, storytelling, collaboration, or support—this book is a reflection of the keys to well-being that you've shared. You make us happier day in and day out. Thank you.

● INTRODUCTION

What makes you happy?

When we asked that question to people around the world, from Mexico to India to the Czech Republic to New Zealand, here is what they shared:

> *Sunshine and hanging out with my friends*

> *Doing nice things for other people*

> *Being outside with the sky above my head*

> *Paragliding, laughing, and eating cake*

> *Cooking something beautiful and enjoying food with family*

> *Helping people and exploring a new environment*

> *Cuddling with my son, Belgian waffles with whipped cream, and the smell of little puppies*

Whether we find them on the water, in the kitchen, or in the arms of a loved one, we all savor moments of happiness. But sometimes these moments feel fleeting, or the sheer weight of the negativity in the world threatens to outweigh them.

Sometimes loneliness, work stress, or worries about the future take over, and it's hard to see anything else.

If you're seeking a deeper sense of happiness in life, there is no shortage of things you can try—or products you can buy. Everything from cold showers to infrared saunas is being touted as the best-kept secret to a life of contentment and bliss.

At the Greater Good Science Center, a nonprofit based at UC Berkeley, our focus is on enduring, research-based practices for happiness and meaning, which we've been sharing in print and online for more than 20 years. The studies that could help us all live better lives could fill libraries, but it's all just words unless we learn how to put them into practice. This workbook takes the best that the science of well-being has to offer and aims to translate it for you to apply to your daily life in a way that feels sustainable and meaningful.

We believe that trying the practices in this workbook could change your life, just as we've witnessed change in the lives of so many of our community members—and in our own.

A LITTLE BACKGROUND

The three of us coauthors, Kira, Jill, and Shuka, were each drawn to the science of well-being for different reasons, and you'll see our perspectives reflected in these pages. Kira has tried many of these practices over the years alongside myriad goals and New Year's resolutions, so she's particularly attuned to the challenges that arise when you try to change your habits. She's now the managing editor of *Greater Good* magazine, having written, edited, and read many, many hundreds of articles on the science of well-being.

Jill was a graduate student in psychology when she first learned about the field of positive psychology—the science of thriving in life—and became interested in its potential for healing or preventing mental illness. She joined *Greater Good* magazine as a writer in 2006 and, since then, has written over 500 articles covering the science of personal and social well-being. Besides communicating the research to others, she applies the lessons learned to her own life, too (and shares them from time to time with her two sons).

Shuka has a background in health care journalism reporting on underrepresented communities in the United States and abroad. Her desire to share solutions-based news, along with her love of storytelling, led her to *Greater Good* in 2018, where she is now the executive producer of audio of the award-winning podcast *The Science of Happiness*. Each episode focuses on research-backed practices (like the ones you'll find in this workbook) to cultivate a happier, more meaningful life.

The science of well-being that we draw from here—much from the field of positive psychology—is unique in a number of ways.

As a field, positive psychology, championed by psychologist Martin Seligman, was born as a complement to psychological research that mostly focused on mental illness and hardship. Its aim was to explore what helps people flourish, rather than merely focusing on what supports us through our psychological struggles.

That led to pioneering studies in gratitude, mindfulness, optimism, and more—but something funny happened. It turned out that positive psychology practices didn't just work for people who were averagely content and wanted to get happier. They could also help those very same people who were struggling—even with very difficult issues, including trauma, chronic illness, or loss—and offer them life-changing tools that focused on their strengths and goodness.

These tools are often bite-sized practices, short enough to do on your lunch break or on a quiet Saturday morning. Many positive psychology experiments test out 10-minute meditations or 20-minute journaling prompts that you can incorporate into your life and that have been found to improve happiness, physical health, and resilience to stress.

Not sure if you want to keep a gratitude journal or meditate? The good news is that there are many different science-based tools at your disposal, which you can experiment with and tweak to fit your needs and interests. This workbook has 21 practices, and you'll find another 80+ on our website Greater Good in Action (ggia.berkeley.edu). We've also consulted with leading well-being researchers to bring you their best tips for success as you continue your journey.

WHAT IS WELL-BEING, ANYWAY?

Happiness is probably one of those things that needs no defining; you know it when you experience it. But scientists, of course, love a good definition—and understanding the different ways they think about well-being may actually help you get clarity on what you're seeking and how you're really doing.

For most researchers, the term *happiness* is interchangeable with "subjective well-being," which is typically measured by asking people about how satisfied they feel with their lives, what level of pleasant and unpleasant emotions they tend to feel, and their sense of meaning and purpose. Recently, some researchers have also explored a notion of the good life that involves *psychological richness*, encompassing curiosity, adventure and exploration, novelty and variety, and an attitude of openness.

At different times in life, you might experience more of some of these types of well-being than others. For example, maybe you recognize that things are generally going well for you in life, but you don't feel so great on a day-to-day basis. Or your life has a lot of fun and enjoyment, but you still feel something is missing.

The practices in this workbook touch on all these different types of well-being.

No matter which type of happiness we're after, though, we should avoid thinking about it as a goal that we're aiming to achieve in the future. If we do, we might fall into the trap of a common happiness myth: anticipating that we'll be happy some day when we finally get X—whether X is a job, a partner, a house, or a kid. Research suggests this just doesn't tend to be true. And while genetics can influence our happiness, it's misleading (not to mention depressing) to believe that some people are happy and some people aren't, and there's nothing we can do about it.[1]

Rather, it helps to think of happiness as a skill or a practice that consists of certain ways of thinking, feeling, and acting. The more we engage in the habits of happiness, the more likely we are to feel happy—and over time, those habits can become more and more automatic and part of our identity.

That doesn't mean we'll feel happy or good all the time, of course. A reliable recipe for unhappiness is to constantly monitor how we feel and judge ourselves when we feel bad or try to push away those uncomfortable feelings. Embracing how we feel in any given moment will ultimately help us feel more content in the long term—a lesson we'll come back to in our chapters on Mindfulness and Self-Compassion.

THE KEYS TO WELL-BEING

This workbook is organized around these happiness habits, the practices and skills that research suggests can help you live a happier, more meaningful life. While we draw from academic research in psychology and other disciplines, many of these practices have a long history across different cultural traditions, from Indigenous cultures to Buddhist practice, reflecting wisdom that has been passed down through generations. The keys to well-being we cover are:

- Connection
- Kindness
- Empathy
- Compassion
- Awe
- Mindfulness
- Gratitude
- Self-Compassion
- Emotion Regulation
- Purpose

Each chapter can stand on its own, so if you don't want to follow the workbook straight through, you're welcome to jump around to topics or themes that speak to you. If your social life needs some nurturing, you might start with Connection or Empathy; if you're struggling more with your thoughts and feelings, you could try Mindfulness or Self-Compassion.

Each chapter is divided into a few sections:

- **The benefits:** What happens when you cultivate these skills? This section explains the evidence suggesting these practices not only make you happier but also benefit your health, relationships, community, and more. Being aware of this research could give you more motivation to set aside time and do the practices.
- **A quiz:** Get an idea of how you're doing currently on these different skills.
- **Two or three practices:** Short, mostly 5- to 20-minute practices that are backed by research, from active listening to appreciating nature to acts of kindness. This workbook offers step-by-step instructions and space to journal or jot down your notes and reflections afterward.
- **Putting it into practice:** Of course, not everything is as simple as following five easy steps. Here you'll find insights from research, psychologists, and students about how to address common challenges, what these skills look like in day-to-day life, and little tips and tricks to spark change.

Some of the richest stories you'll read in this workbook come from our *Science of Happiness* podcast guests, who took the time to try out these practices and share how it went—along with different variations they tested, pitfalls they encountered, and takeaways for their own lives. You'll hear from Aaron Harvey, who chose a life of kindness and activism after being wrongfully incarcerated for months; Diana Gameros, who found awe in Mexico after 16 years of being separated from her homeland and her family; and former U.S. Surgeon General Vivek Murthy, who grew up feeling lonely and is now working to counter the loneliness epidemic in today's society.

JOIN THE MOVEMENT

In the fall of 2014, our team launched a new online course called The Science of Happiness. It started with two instructors (Emiliana Simon-Thomas and Dacher Keltner), a slew of videos filmed in our office conference room, and the hope that curious learners might be interested in research and practices to help them live happier, more meaningful lives.

We weren't quite prepared for the response. That first semester, over 125,000 students signed up. Over the next 10 years, we would register upwards of three-quarters of a million in total from more than 190 countries, from Pakistan to Iceland to Ghana. According to surveys students took throughout the course, learning about the science of happiness for 10 weeks helped them experience more positive emotions, less stress and loneliness, and a stronger sense of connectedness to humanity.

Around the world, people like our Science of Happiness students are applying the science of well-being to their everyday lives to feel better, improve their relationships, and get more out of their precious time on earth—and its insights have spread to schools, workplaces, governments, and beyond.

We hope you'll join us, and them, on the journey.

Based on community feedback, we know it's not always easy: We hear that you're tired and stressed, and you don't want yet another obligation to squeeze between commuting and child care and reading the news. We recognize the deep-rooted injustices that permeate our society and workplaces, which won't change overnight and which no single one of us can fix. We hear that you need support, and lightness, and hope.

The practices in this book offer you the opportunity for positive moments, to ponder some ideas you might not have thought of before and have some enjoyable and eye-opening interactions with your friends and family. And, hopefully, you'll start seeing the little shifts in your life that you are seeking.

If you'd like to stay in touch with the latest science we're sharing at the Greater Good Science Center, you can find us at greatergood.berkeley.edu and find new practices on Greater Good in Action (ggia.berkeley.edu). You can also listen to our *Science of Happiness* podcast wherever you listen to your podcasts.

No matter how you arrived here, we are *happy* that you picked up this workbook. There is something courageous, and hopeful, in believing that change is possible and taking steps to make it happen. Let's get started!

The Science of Happiness
Workbook

Chapter 1
Connection

When Vivek Murthy was a child, he'd wake every morning filled with a deep sense of dread. He would get out of bed, get dressed, eat breakfast, and feel the tightness in his chest expand through his body as he sat in the backseat of his parents' car on the way to elementary school.

"I didn't want to be alone on the playground," Murthy says. "Or alone when they asked people to partner up in class on exercises. And I certainly dreaded walking into the cafeteria each day, not knowing if there would be somebody to sit next to. That pain ran deep. And that sense of deep loneliness stayed with me for many, many years."

Murthy went on to study at Yale and Harvard, become a physician, and then become the first surgeon general of the United States of Indian descent under Presidents Obama, Trump, and Biden.

Murthy had a perfect, accomplished life—from the outside. On the inside, he still felt lonely.

"Feeling socially connected isn't what's on your resume," says Murthy. "It's about how you perceive yourself and how you measure the world, and if you tend to look more at the darkness or at the light."

Murthy began to study loneliness, both his own and its greater societal impacts. He found that loneliness was epidemic—and not just in the United

States. "In my conversations with health care leaders from other countries, I really saw that many other nations were experiencing very high rates of loneliness."

In his research, Murphy discovered that loneliness is less about being alone and more about feeling dissatisfied with the connections we have. When we are chronically lonely, over time we experience an erosion of self-esteem. We come to believe that we're lonely because we're not likable, we're broken in some way. We tend to become ashamed and turn inward.

We also get sick.[1] Research finds that loneliness actually activates the same brain networks as physical pain,[2] and it can lead to weakened immune function,[3] increased levels of inflammation,[4] and an increased risk of heart disease, stroke,[5] cancer,[6] diabetes,[7] dementia, depression, and anxiety.

But Murthy was most struck by the data on longevity.

"The degree to which our life is shortened is similar for loneliness as it is for smoking 15 cigarettes a day," he explains.

These health effects are signals that our bodies send us when we're lacking something we need for survival: healthy human connection. "And in that sense, it's very similar to hunger, to thirst," says Murthy.

The Office of the Surgeon General has a decades-long legacy of addressing smoking, obesity, and sedentary living, yet Murthy realized that loneliness had not been on their radar at all as an important public health issue.

So, after decades of struggling with his own loneliness in secret, Murthy vowed to speak up and bring more connection into his life and into the folds of society.

THE BENEFITS OF CONNECTION

When Harvard researchers began a study on longevity and well-being in the 1930s, they didn't know how long it would run or what they would find.[8] They began tracking men from different neighborhoods in the Boston area, asking about their health, income, employment, and marital status. The men also filled out questionnaires and participated in interviews throughout the years to reveal their inner lives—their fears, hopes, disappointments, accomplishments, regrets, life satisfaction, and much more.

After more than eight decades, during which people of other genders and backgrounds were added to the study, the researchers came to a fairly provocative conclusion: While work accomplishments and healthy behaviors contribute to well-being, they aren't what matter most. Instead, warm, positive relationships are the key to a happier, healthier life.[9]

The centrality of our relationships to well-being is backed up by many other long-term studies, including those looking at diverse groups of people in terms of age, race, ethnicity, and gender.[10, 11, 12] It holds true in introverts and extraverts alike.[13] Strong relationships are what seem to set apart very happy people—the top 10%—from the rest.[14]

Nurturing our social connections is a powerful way to increase happiness. In one German study, people rated how satisfied they were with life and then provided ideas for how they could increase their happiness over time. Some chose activities that boosted their social connection, like seeing friends and family more or volunteering—while others chose goals that were more individual, like losing weight or finding a better job. A year later, those who'd chosen social goals and followed through on them were significantly happier. Those who'd successfully accomplished individual goals were not.[15]

On a moment-to-moment basis, research finds that we are happiest when we are with other people we know care about us—compared to doing any other types of activities.[16] We get a warm burst of feeling when we cuddle with our kids, share worries with a best friend, or make love to our romantic partner. Even when relationships require effort and hard work, they can still bring happiness to our lives overall, because those close ties provide meaning in life.[17]

Whether considering our friends, family, neighbors, colleagues, or larger communities, we benefit when our social connections are strong.

> "Indigenous contemplative practices reorient the focus to the larger systems of relationships that humans are only part of, bringing equal emphasis to self, community, and environment through keen awareness of relational networks" —Yuria Celidwen, Indigenous scholar[18]

THE ROOTS OF CONNECTION

Why is social connection so important? The reasons probably lie in early human evolution, when having others to rely on helped us stay safe from outside threats. Throughout history, the worst punishments included banishment from the tribe and solitary confinement, because social connection was so important for us to survive. That need explains why our brains are so exquisitely wired for connection, helping us to pay close attention to other people, empathize, and experience positive feelings when in a relationship.[19]

"To the extent that we can characterize evolution as designing our modern brains, this is what our brains were wired for: reaching out to and interacting with others," writes neuroscientist Matthew Lieberman in his book *Social*.[20]

From the time we are young, we require connection to a parental figure to survive, and those early bonds can be crucial for setting the stage for well-being. Forming what researchers call a *secure attachment* with our caregivers—knowing we are loved and can safely be who we are—has all kinds of benefits later on, including improved social and emotional skills, cognitive functioning, physical health, and mental health.[21]

Still, even the problems that come with less secure attachments with caregivers can be overcome if we can develop more secure attachments to others in our lives. We may just need to look beyond our families of origin to find the warm, supportive relationships that help us thrive.

HOW DIFFERENT TYPES OF RELATIONSHIPS MAKE US HAPPIER

When it comes to happiness, many of us minimize the importance of social ties with people *outside* of our immediate families. But those relationships can provide a sense of meaning and belonging, while helping us meet the challenges of life with more joy and resilience.

Friendships, in particular, can be not only fun and enjoyable, but also help buffer us against stress and provide outlets for processing difficult emotions.[22,23] As one long-term study of mostly European New Zealanders found, being socially connected in our younger years predicts our happiness as an adult better than doing well at school.[24] And those childhood friendships can even bring us health benefits—like reduced blood pressure and a healthy body weight.[25]

Putting effort into our friendships can have a big payoff, as one student from our Science of Happiness course found: "The energy I put into the world when I made an intention to have friends who were authentic and caring humans like myself was met 100%," says Talib Jasir from New Jersey. "My attachment to those relationships has changed my life and most importantly . . . has created a great deal of happiness that I had never thought possible."

It's also important to consider our looser social ties—the people we interact with in our workplaces, schools, neighborhoods, or communities at large. They, too, matter for our well-being.

In fact, one Canadian study found that people are happier on days when they have more interactions with acquaintances and strangers.[26] Another study in Finland found that people live longer if they have a larger number of loose social ties, apart from whether or not they have close, intimate ties.[27]

Even connecting with strangers can make us happier. In one well-known study, people in Illinois were asked to start up a conversation with a stranger during their normal commute, or keep to themselves or do whatever they would normally do. Beforehand, they rated how happy they were and how much they desired solitude. Those who engaged in conversation ended up happier at the end of their commute—even if they predicted that they'd enjoy their solitude more than socializing.[28] If that sounds interesting to you, be sure to try the Small Talk practice below!

As researcher Hanne Collins says, "The more you can broaden your social portfolio and reach out to people you talk to less frequently—like an acquaintance, an old friend, a coworker, or even a stranger in the grocery store—the more it could have really positive benefits for your well-being."

REFLECT

In which areas of life are your connections strong? In which areas of life would you like to feel more connected?

_____
_____
_____
_____
_____

CONNECTED COMMUNITIES

While having a sense of belonging and connection with others is important to flourishing, loneliness (its opposite) is one of the prime happiness killers. That's why it's important to create equitable communities where social connection flourishes and people know that they belong. Too many of us face discrimination or social isolation because of our age, ethnicity, race, gender, or sexual orientation, and that's bound to increase all of the ills of loneliness.

When we feel more connected to each other, in large and small ways, we help create a society that is more trusting, compassionate, and loving—which, in turn, supports personal happiness. For all of these reasons, it behooves us to find ways to develop positive social connections, with both people we know and those we don't yet know. If you want to learn more about how to nurture connection in your own life, read on.

HOW CONNECTED ARE YOU?

Before we offer you connection practices to try out, we'd like to give you the opportunity to reflect on your own feelings of connectedness.[29] If you'd like, you can revisit these questions later to see if taking steps to connect made a difference.

	Strongly disagree	Disagree	Neutral	Agree	Strongly agree
I feel distant from people.	5	4	3	2	1
I feel understood by the people I know.	1	2	3	4	5
My friends feel like family.	1	2	3	4	5
I feel close to people.	1	2	3	4	5
I feel comfortable in the presence of strangers.	1	2	3	4	5
I am able to relate to my peers.	1	2	3	4	5
I feel like an outsider.	5	4	3	2	1
I see people as friendly and approachable.	1	2	3	4	5
I fit in well in new situations.	1	2	3	4	5
I find myself actively involved in people's lives.	1	2	3	4	5

Quick scoring guide: 10–30 = Low; 31–40 = Medium; 41–50 = High

CONNECTION PRACTICES

As part of his efforts to connect more deeply with others, and as an exercise for our *Science of Happiness* podcast, Murthy reached out to an old friend living abroad, and asked him to share something good that happened to him that day—and Murthy listened. They ended up making it a weekly practice, using a video call so they could see each other.

"What's really important is that we were fully present with one another," Murthy says. "That means making eye contact, putting away our phones and other distractions. It means giving the other person the gift of your full attention, listening deeply, and also asking thoughtful questions."

Murthy would often enter those conversations stressed and uncentered. As U.S. surgeon general, he was always in and out of meetings and also feeling like a bad father to his young children because he was so stretched for time. But as soon as he started talking, he would feel things settle inside of him. "It felt like time expanded," he says.

In a world that is so oriented around taking action, Murthy realized we can forget just how impactful it is to pause and have the experience of listening deeply to someone else.

"Sometimes the power of our presence in itself can be deeply healing," Murthy says. "These conversations were an opportunity to focus on what was good, on the positive, and on what I had to be grateful for. I needed to do that more consciously."

The practice Murthy tried for our podcast is called Capitalizing on Positive Events, and research suggests that it can improve your relationships—and help the other person feel good.[30, 31] You can try it for yourself:

 PRACTICE #1: CAPITALIZING ON POSITIVE EVENTS
Time: 5 minutes

Read the steps of this practice, based on research by Shelly Gable, and then plan out a time to try it.

Ask a friend, family member, colleague, romantic partner, or other acquaintance to tell you about a good thing that happened to them today. It doesn't matter what type of event or how important it was, as long as they feel comfortable discussing it.

As they share, listen and try to respond actively and constructively, meaning that you:

- **To the best of your ability, make good eye contact.** This shows that they have your full attention and that you are interested in what they have to say.
- **Express positive emotion.** This could be smiling, nodding, or even cheering (if appropriate!).
- **Make enthusiastic comments.** For example, "That sounds great," "You must be so excited," or "Your hard work is definitely paying off."
- **Ask open-ended questions to find out more about the positive parts of the event.** Questions about who, what, when, where, or why can help sustain your conversation. For example, if the person tells you about receiving recognition at work for a project they completed, you could ask for more details about the project, what aspects of the project they feel especially proud of, or how it felt to be recognized.
- **Comment on the positive implications and potential benefits of the event.** For example, "I bet this means you have a better chance of getting a promotion this year."

One strategy is to pick a specific aspect of the event that sticks out to you and begin by commenting on that: "You seem really happy about what your boss said—tell me more." Or "It must have been satisfying to do so well on something you worked so hard for."

Many people, when they first hear about this exercise, worry that their responses will sound phony or scripted. However, once they start, they tend to report that it feels natural and easy to do.

Make a plan: With whom could you try Capitalizing on Positive Events? List some ideas for when and where you could make it happen this week. Come back and journal about how it went!

Who:
_____
_____

When:
_____
_____

How did it go? How did they respond to your interest? Did you feel more connected?
_____
_____
_____
_____

 PRACTICE #2: FEELING CONNECTED
Time: 5 minutes

This is a writing practice that research suggests can help you generate the warm, positive feelings of connection—and boost your kindness too.[32]

Bring to mind someone to whom you feel very close. Who is this person?

_____

Think of a time when you felt especially close and connected to them. This could be a time you had a meaningful conversation, gave or received support, experienced a great loss or success together, or witnessed a historic moment together. Then, write a short paragraph describing it in detail: What happened? Where? When? How did you feel? In particular, consider the ways in which this experience made you feel bonded to the other person.

_____
_____
_____
_____
_____
_____
_____
_____

 PRACTICE #3: SMALL TALK
Time: 10 minutes

Read the steps of this practice now, and then plan out a time to try it.

In our everyday lives, we routinely spend time around strangers but don't always strike up conversations with them. This exercise invites you to make a connection rather than remaining in solitude.

Whether during your commute, in a waiting room or an elevator, or in line for coffee, have a conversation with a new person today. Try to make a connection. Find out something interesting about them, and share something about yourself. The longer the conversation, the better. Your goal is to try to get to know the person.

Although people are probably more willing to talk than you expect, it's important to be sensitive if you sense that your conversation partner doesn't want to engage. If they do seem interested, here are some tips for a good conversation:

- **Ask questions related to your immediate context.** At a grocery store, you might ask, "What are you going to make with that?"
- **Have some go-to questions.** For example, "What do you do for fun?" or "Where are you from?"
- **Leverage your knowledge of news or current events.** You might ask, "Did you hear about the couple who won the lottery? What would you do if you won?"
- **Explore their interests.** This tends to work well if you seem to have something in common. For example, "Are you on your way to yoga? What's your favorite type of class?"
- **Ask follow-up questions.** Rather than flitting from topic to topic, go deeper into the conversation.

Make a plan: Who could you try Small Talk with (e.g., a neighbor, a passenger on the bus, a work contact)? Write down a few conversation starters and ideas for when and where you could do it this week. Come back and journal about how it went!

Who:
_____

When:
_____

Potential questions:

How did it go? How did they respond to you starting a conversation? How did you feel afterward?

PUTTING CONNECTION INTO PRACTICE

As long as we don't live on a desert island, people are all around us. That means that we have plenty of opportunities to try to connect. It can be messy at times, or awkward, or painful, but that is all part of being human. In those moments of connection, we may find a deep sense of fulfillment, meaning, and belonging.

OVERCOMING LONELINESS

Among all the ways loneliness hurts us, there's one that's particularly cruel: It can perpetuate our isolation and keep us distant from others by influencing how we think and act.

"Loneliness, unfortunately, carries stigma with it. People who feel lonely often are ashamed to admit it," says Murthy. "They think it's equivalent to admitting that they are not likable or that they're socially insufficient in some way."

In one study in Germany and the U.K., researchers found that when people felt lonely, they had more negative social interactions, possibly because they acted in ways that made socializing less fulfilling than it could have been.[33]

"Loneliness predisposes people to approach social interactions with cynicism, distrust, and an expectation of rejection and betrayal [which] might in turn negatively affect other people's behavior towards them," write researchers Olga Stavrova and Dongning Ren.[34]

This makes the solutions to loneliness complicated. Unfortunately, Stavrova and Ren's study found that spending time with other people won't necessarily make you feel better when you're lonely. Instead, the antidotes to loneliness may be more inward-looking, overcoming the inner soundtrack that makes it harder for us to connect with others. One review study found that the best strategy is to question automatic negative thoughts that might tell us that we're to blame for feeling bad, we're too needy, or no one wants to be our friend.[35]

Simple self-care practices, like taking care of our sleep and exercise, or doing certain types of meditation, have also been found to reduce loneliness.[36, 37, 38] And it helps to recognize that loneliness is a common struggle. A survey in early 2024 found that 30% of U.S. adults feel lonely at least every week, and that number may be even higher among parents, Hispanic and Black adults, and people with low incomes. The lonely are less alone than we think.

Alongside the inner work of coping with loneliness,[39, 40] the usual tips for making friends and bolstering connections apply. There are endless ways to do this, but here are a few of the tips we find most impactful:

- **Look for connection at three levels.** Intimate (partner or spouse), relational (circle of friends), and collective (community). "There is a sense of connection we experience, even with strangers, that's very valuable, that makes you feel like you're part of something bigger," says Murthy.

- **Practice kindness for others.** Loneliness can keep us focused on ourselves. If you go into an interaction trying to do good for others, you may feel less worried about how you're being perceived. Stay tuned for the Kindness chapter!
- **Reach out and have a conversation with a friend today.** Catch up, laugh or joke around, offer support and listening, or give them a compliment. Research suggests that this one small interaction can make you feel more connected and less stressed at the end of your day.[41] And bonus points if you do a phone or video call rather than text or email—it can make you feel even more connected and happy.[42]

GETTING CLOSER

Relationships are about quality as well as quantity. So how can we feel close and connected in the relationships that we have already?

Attachment styles are our ways of relating to others that we learned in childhood. Simply having knowledge of them is helpful in recognizing patterns within ourselves and others that can disrupt connection—especially in romantic relationships. They tend to come in four types:

- **Secure attachment:** You are confident and able to establish intimacy, and you generally trust people in relationships.
- **Anxious attachment:** You are worried and preoccupied about closeness. You fear being abandoned and tend to cling to others.
- **Avoidant attachment:** Closeness feels uncomfortable, and you tend to withdraw from others. You may come off as aloof and distant or have trouble trusting others.
- **Disorganized attachment:** You show conflicting behaviors that sometimes look like anxiety and sometimes look like avoidance.[43]

If we have an insecure attachment style, there's good news: Positive experiences in relationships as adults may be able to help us heal. Receiving more gratitude from a partner can help ease anxious attachment, whereas activities that foster intimacy—like deep conversations and partner yoga—may help reduce avoidant attachment.[44, 45]

OPENING UP

No matter what your attachment style, relationships can bring discomfort and vulnerability. When we open ourselves up to others, we risk being judged—or getting hurt.

But research suggests the opposite of these fears.[46] In fact, you endear yourself to others when you share intimacies with them, as long as you don't overshare or use vulnerability to manipulate someone.[47]

"In order for connection to happen, we have to allow ourselves to be seen, really seen," says Brené Brown in her TED talk *The Power of Vulnerability.* According to her research, the people who have a strong sense of love and belonging are the ones who embrace vulnerability—who say "I love you" first, who invest in a relationship that could end, who put themselves out there when they might get hurt.

"They believed that what made them vulnerable made them beautiful. They didn't talk about vulnerability being comfortable . . . they just talked about it being necessary," says Brown.[48]

REFLECT

What is your attachment style(s)? How do you feel about being vulnerable with others? Do you find it hard to trust people?

While Murthy served as U.S. surgeon general, his investigations into loneliness led to his book, *Together: The Healing Power of Human Connection in a Sometimes Lonely World.*

In his personal life, Murthy noticed that his mood lifted thanks to weekly chats with his friend. Their conversations were brief, sometimes no more than 15 minutes, but the impact on his emotional state and sense of peace lasted for hours afterward. He felt more optimistic about the world and less weighed down by its challenges. He felt a boost of physical energy, as well. That brief amount of time connecting with his friend, done consistently, rejuvenated him.

Murthy soon understood that these connective moments could be found anywhere: a compassionate greeting from the barista at a coffee shop, a kind comment from a work colleague, a warm hello on the elevator. When Murthy was fully present, fully listening, he was able to derive a lot from these short interactions—they were all opportunities to connect.

"I've come to realize that we evolved to be social creatures, that we were meant to be together and that we are truly interdependent," says Murthy. "And when you understand that, then this larger mission to make us a more connected community and help us build more connected lives is not an effort to transform us into something that we are not, it's an effort to return us to who we naturally are."

Chapter 2

Kindness

Aaron Harvey had more than his share of reasons to harbor bitterness toward others.

Growing up in a high-crime neighborhood in southeast San Diego, California, he was stopped and handcuffed by police officers at age 11, simply because he resembled another Black boy who was suspected of a crime.

At 26, he was arrested and charged in connection with a series of gang shootings that he wasn't involved in, just because he was documented as a gang member based on his social media posts.

He spent the next 8 months in jail, on a $1.1 million bail, looking at 56 years to life. His lawyer recommended he sign a plea deal to do 19 years in prison.

"I was tired—jail is really meant to break a person's mind and spirit," says Harvey. "I felt like I had every right to hate people." But his father reminded him that instead of hate, he could be inspired by the examples of Malcolm X and Martin Luther King Jr.—and turn to a life of kindness.

Harvey didn't take the plea deal, and he was eventually released. Inspired by his father, he started looking for opportunities to be kind.

Six years later, Harvey tried the Random Acts of Kindness practice for our *Science of Happiness* podcast: five kind things for five people, in one day. First thing in the morning, he drove to his local Starbucks to buy his mother a coffee and a bite to eat for breakfast—a small act to thank her for all her support helping watch his young daughter while he studied to get his bachelor's degree.

But things took a different turn.

When he arrived at the coffee shop, he saw a man standing outside the door, looking in need of some help. So Harvey offered to buy him coffee and a meal.

"I ended up buying him the Starbucks and as I was walking away, something dawned on me," Harvey says. "No, I'm not doing it this way." He turned around and walked back to the man. "Hey, I'm sorry. What's your name?"

"Ronald."

"I'm Aaron, nice to meet you."

In the past, Harvey had bought meals for people who had looked like they could use help, but he had never stopped to ask their names. "I never took the time to actually get to know that person or to talk to them," Harvey says.

They struck up a conversation, and Harvey learned that Ronald was about to move into a new apartment that day.

Harvey offered to help him move—he had a friend who owned a moving company, and could borrow his truck. Ronald gratefully accepted his offer.

"That made me happy because it brought him some type of peace, some type of joy, of accomplishment, that he was moving up in the ladder of life," Harvey says. "By getting to know a person, even if it's just for like two minutes, there's much more impact that you can have on their life."

Four hours later, while Harvey was wrapping up helping Ronald move, he got a phone call from a good friend who was stranded on the freeway with a flat tire. So he got in the car, headed toward his friend, and helped fix his tire.

Harvey ended up doing all five random acts of kindness that day—except for the one he intended to do.

"I never made it back to my mom to get her breakfast," says Harvey. "But that [day] made me look at my life [like] more of a 'glass half full.'"

THE BENEFITS OF KINDNESS

The human urge to be kind has deep roots. Children as young as 18 months will go out of their way to try to help someone in need.[1] If they see someone drop an object that they can't reach, children will make an effort to pick it up and return it. And children as young as 2 years old appear to be happier when they give to others than when they receive something for themselves.[2]

Examples of kindness are abundant in everyday life. We may open the door for someone whose arms are full of groceries or offer to help our partner do the dishes. We may give a colleague our full attention, stop to help a stranded driver, or donate to charity. When observed in their everyday lives, people around the world practice kindness regularly, often without much forethought.[3]

And then there's the kindness that Harvey offered, beyond an ordinary act of generosity—getting to know someone's story, going the extra mile to help out. Though that kind of altruism can certainly make you happier, research suggests that even small acts of kindness can carry significant benefits, for people on both sides of them—enough to make you seek out more ways to be kind. Here are some research-backed reasons why kindness is more than just a nice idea: It's actually good for you, your relationships, and the world.

KINDNESS MAKES YOU HAPPIER

Whatever way we practice it, kindness is its own reward. Even if we aren't thinking about our own interests when practicing kindness, it often brings us an increased sense of meaning and closeness to others, which in turn makes us happier.

In one study, researcher Sonja Lyubomirsky and her colleagues asked a group of mostly white or Asian American people to do three kind acts in one day either for another person (like making dinner for a friend) or for humanity in general (e.g., picking up street garbage). Others were asked to do three nice things to make themselves happy (e.g., take a longer lunch break at work) or just keep track of their activities, once a week for 4 weeks. People doing acts of kindness reported being much happier over time than those in the other groups, and this bump in happiness lasted 2 weeks after the experiment was over.[4]

Analyzing many studies together, researchers find that your age, gender, or education don't seem to matter—practicing kind acts will almost always benefit your well-being, whether you are a middle school girl in Hong Kong or a man in a Chinese prison.[5, 6]

Giving to others can make us happier when it involves spending money, too.[7, 8] In one experiment, Canadian adult students were given money to buy a goodie bag filled with treats and were told it would be either for themselves or for an anonymous sick child. According to surveys, those who were assigned to buy treats for the child were much happier than those who spent money on themselves.[9] Another study found similar results when people had an opportunity to spend money to protect others during the COVID-19 pandemic—during a time of uncertainty, when you might expect folks to be focused on their own needs.[10]

Paradoxically, whenever we focus on trying to make others feel good, it tends to make us feel better—more so than aiming to make ourselves feel good directly.[11] This could be because doing something for others takes the focus off of ourselves and our own troubles.

REFLECT

Think about a recent time you practiced kindness toward someone else. What did you do, and how did it make you feel?

_____
_____
_____
_____

KINDNESS IMPROVES YOUR HEALTH

Being kind to others can improve your health too.[12] If we spend money to help others, it tends to lower our blood pressure, which improves our cardiovascular functioning.[13] People who volunteer tend to experience fewer aches and pains, better overall physical health, and less depression[14]; older people who volunteer or regularly help friends or relatives live significantly longer lives than those who don't.[15, 16]

Why is that? No one knows for sure. It could be that being kind affects our health indirectly by making us feel better about ourselves and our lives. It may help boost our sense of competence, distract us from stressors, or help us be more connected to others. Whatever the reasons, kindness both *feels* good and *does* good.

KINDNESS IMPROVES OUR RELATIONSHIPS— AND OUR WORLD

As Lyubomirsky writes in her book *The How of Happiness*, "Being kind and generous leads you to perceive others more positively and more charitably," which makes kindness act as a kind of social glue. The way kindness binds us together suggests it could be an evolutionary adaptation, designed to help us not only find a partner, but live together more smoothly in cooperative societies.

We can be kind in our own household, in our own city, and ultimately toward the whole world. Science of Happiness student Cyndi Barron from Canada found that, even though she lives in a large city, practicing kindness toward strangers led to "unexpected small shocks of recognition and gratefulness," adding to her sense of commonality.

"It makes me feel good to know that it really doesn't take much to reach out beyond the barriers between strangers," she says. "It makes me feel light and happy."

Luckily, kindness can be contagious. Witnessing unexpected acts of kindness—like someone delivering food to a homeless person or helping a visually impaired person cross a busy intersection—can give us a sense of *moral elevation*, a warm and uplifting feeling. In turn, that feeling makes us more likely to volunteer our time and offer help. Even everyday kind acts on the news or on TV can inspire us to want to pay it forward by acting kind ourselves.[17] This could help kindness spread within a community, creating a sort of *virtuous circle* that benefits everyone.

So, if you're curious to try it out yourself and see how kindness can enhance your life, read on.

HOW KIND ARE YOU?

Before we offer you kindness practices to try out, we'd like to give you the opportunity to reflect on your own behaviors and attitudes around kindness.[18] If you like, you can revisit these questions later to see if deliberately practicing kindness made a difference.

	Strongly disagree	Disagree	Neutral	Agree	Strongly agree
Helping friends and family is one of the great joys in life.	1	2	3	4	5
I try to offer my help with any activities my community or school groups are carrying out.	1	2	3	4	5
I try to cheer up people who appear unhappy.	1	2	3	4	5
When given the opportunity, I enjoy aiding others who are in need.	1	2	3	4	5
I help people when they ask.	1	2	3	4	5
I donate time or money to charities every month.	1	2	3	4	5

	Strongly disagree	Disagree	Neutral	Agree	Strongly agree
I feel at peace with myself when I have helped others.	1	2	3	4	5
I would let someone in a rush cut ahead of me in line.	1	2	3	4	5
I will listen to a friend's problems as long as they need.	1	2	3	4	5
I like to make other people feel happy.	1	2	3	4	5

Quick scoring guide: 10–30 = Low; 31–40 = Medium; 41–50 = High

KINDNESS PRACTICES

PRACTICE #1: RANDOM ACTS OF KINDNESS

Time: 10 minutes

1. Think of five people you might see today, including some you know (like family members) and some who are unfamiliar (e.g., a store clerk).
2. List each person, and then write one thing you could do to brighten their day. It could be as simple as a friendly compliment or a few words of encouragement; you could pay for a stranger's coffee, pick up litter, help a friend with a chore, or provide a meal to a person in need.
3. Get started: Say something kind, or send a friendly message to someone right now!

Examples:

My neighbor: I could bring her a gift, like food or some flowers.

My colleague at work: I could see if he needs help with anything.

1. _____
2. _____
3. _____
4. _____
5. _____

If you said or sent something friendly or kind just now, to whom did you say it and what did you say?

Did you notice any feelings or thoughts that came up while you were thinking of kind things to do or friendly things to say or send?

Which of the kind things from your list could you plan to do today?

At the end of the day: For each act, write down what you did in at least one or two sentences; for more of a happiness boost, also write down how it made you feel.

_____
_____
_____
_____
_____
_____
_____
_____
_____

PRACTICE #2: GIFT OF TIME

Time: Varies

Certain acts of kindness entail gifts of money or goods, but, in this exercise, the gift you're giving is your time. Research suggests that this practice can boost your happiness up to 1 month later.[19]

1. List a few people to whom you could offer a Gift of Time this week, and some ideas for when you could make it happen. It might mean doing something with them (in person or virtually) or something for them on your own, like cooking their favorite dish for dinner.

Name	What will you do for them?	When?

2. Give these gifts of your time. Spend as much time as needed to do the favor well and do not take any shortcuts. You might even consider taking off your watch or putting your phone away.
3. If you did something for them on your own, do not tell the recipient of your gift how much time you spent. Let the gift speak for itself.
4. What was the experience like? How did you feel, and (if applicable) what did the other person feel? What did you learn?

"You can be kind. You can be generous. I think there's this narrative that generosity is a luxury sport. It's our human right to be kind and to be loving. And you don't need material things to do that."
—Nipun Mehta, founder of ServiceSpace

PUTTING KINDNESS INTO PRACTICE

While research suggests that kindness comes naturally to humans—and may even have an evolutionary basis—many different things can get in the way of us acting on our kinder instincts in our everyday lives. That means you might be missing out on opportunities to be generous and helpful that could benefit you and others.

THE AWKWARDNESS OF KINDNESS

We may be stifling our own kindness based on mistaken beliefs about other people. In one study, people in Chicago and Austin underestimated the impact of being kind. Whether they were giving someone a hot chocolate or cupcake, or writing them a nice note, they didn't realize how happy their kindness would make the other person feel.[20]

Maybe we worry that people won't appreciate it if we're kind to them—especially strangers whose reactions could be hard to predict—or that people will think we're weird or pushy or condescending in some way.

Even giving someone a compliment can be fraught—research suggests that we think the people we compliment will feel more bothered and uncomfortable, and less positive, than they actually do.[21] These false assumptions are based on us feeling anxious and thinking that we're not that adept at giving compliments.

Of course, the responses to our kindness won't always be positive. Science of Happiness student Teri Grander felt she struck out with her acts of kindness. She tried to help a stranger who fell, but they pushed her; she brought a coworker a cup of coffee, but got weird looks from her colleagues; and she paid for a boy's candy, but was embarrassed by all the attention it brought her. Meanwhile, other students talked about cultural norms in their countries that meant their acts of kindness were met with hurt pride, suspicion, or irritation. While this chapter offers lots of ideas and examples of acts of kindness, you ultimately know best what the people around you might appreciate.

> "The most important part of the random acts of kindness is to not have an outcome in mind. Just do it because you want to, because you think it's a good thing to do. " —Science of Happiness student Anita Bauer Arnold from California

If you aren't worried about the reaction to your kindness, maybe planning acts of kindness and going out and executing them simply feels unnatural to you. The morning Aaron Harvey woke up and decided to buy his mother coffee as an act of kindness, he certainly felt that way.

"It definitely felt weird in the beginning," Harvey says. "The difficulty of me going out and saying, 'OK, I'm intentionally going to do these five things,' it felt a little performative for me, or ungenuine."

Some Science of Happiness students had this experience, and some decided not to plan acts of kindness at all—but rather to mindfully pay attention to the kind acts they were already doing.

If it's helpful, you can think about these practices as strengthening your kindness muscles, until kindness just becomes a way of life for you.

DO YOU HAVE TIME AND ENERGY TO BE KIND?

Simply feeling too busy can also be a barrier to kindness. In studies by Daniel Batson and John Darley, when people walked by someone slumped over on a sidewalk, whether they helped or not depended on a single factor: if they were running late.[22] The great irony of this study, and probably the reason why it's so famous, is that they were seminary students running late to give a talk on the Good Samaritan, a parable from the Bible about helping a traveler who lies helpless on the side of the road. Participants were six times more likely to help when they felt they had the time.

"When we feel time-poor, we're less kind. We spend less time helping other people," says researcher Cassie Mogilner Holmes, who found that spending 10 to 30 minutes doing something kind for another person makes us feel we have *more* time, compared to spending that time on ourselves.[23]

Seeing opportunities for kindness does take a little attention and awareness, and perhaps even some slowing down. But our acts of kindness don't have to be grand gestures, and they don't have to take lots of time.

CAN YOU STILL HELP OTHERS WHEN YOU NEED HELP YOURSELF?

Even if we're not too busy, maybe we feel we have too many of our own problems to be kind to others. But research finds that, even when we're struggling in life, kindness can be a balm.

In a 2022 study, people in the Midwestern United States experiencing depression or anxiety symptoms who practiced random acts of kindness for 5 weeks reduced their symptoms as much or more than those who planned social activities or practiced combating negative thought patterns—both techniques used to treat depression and anxiety.[24] Plus, kindness gave them an added bonus: a greater sense of belonging and social connectedness.

"The nice thing about doing acts of kindness is that you don't even have to enjoy doing them, you don't have to *try* to experience positive feelings," says researcher Jennifer Cheavens. "Kind acts help you get outside of yourself a little and engage [your sense of] meaning." In other words, kindness can be good medicine for what ails us—even if we don't think it will be.

This was the case for one of our Science of Happiness students, who was having a hard week waiting on a medical diagnosis. "Having this practice of Random Acts of Kindness on my mind distracted me from my own plight. I was able to shift my thinking towards others and focused on helping people or just being extra nice and open to strangers," says Wiebke Light from California. "It made my own difficulties seem less difficult and the world appeared a bit smaller and more intimate. Everyone is struggling, but together we can make the suffering and struggling less difficult."

Of course, there are times when we are truly overloaded, and the challenge is in setting boundaries on our own kindness and generosity—performing an act of kindness toward yourself, that will allow you to keep being kind to others in the long term.[25] Self-kindness is crucial, and we'll discuss that more in the chapter on self-compassion.

"Before I can give to those in need," says social entrepreneur Isaac Addae, "I have to sustain the things that sustain me."

REFLECT

What are your barriers to kindness? What makes kindness challenging for you at times?

_____
_____
_____
_____
_____
_____

HOW TO EXPAND YOUR KINDNESS

If you're already a kindness expert, one consideration you might want to reflect on is who the recipients of your kindness typically are. Although there are some mixed findings,[26] one study found that kindness to acquaintances and strangers makes us just as happy as kindness to friends and family.[27] This was the case for adults from over two dozen countries—from the United States and Brazil to the U.K. and South Africa—who performed acts of kindness daily for a week, from helping a neighbor to writing a thank you card to paying for someone's movie ticket.

This is relevant when we consider kindness to people who are different from us, who aren't part of those we call our own community. One study in

South Korea found that coworkers are less kind to each other when they have less in common. In workplaces with more diversity in terms of gender and education, people were less likely to help each other with work problems, show genuine concern and courtesy, and be welcoming to new employees.[28] This likely arises from our tendency to connect with people who are similar to us, and the biases that result from it. So how do we overcome this and create a world that is truly kind to all?

Find shared identity. One way is to try to focus on the things we have in common with others, however ordinary they might be, despite our differences. A U.K. study found that soccer fans were less likely to help an injured jogger if that jogger was wearing the jersey of a rival team.[29] However, when participants were reminded of their larger, more general identity as soccer fans, they were just as likely to help a rival fan as they were to help someone rooting for their favorite team—though less likely to help someone who wasn't wearing a soccer jersey at all.

While not everyone is a soccer fan, of course, we all have identities, traits, or experiences that can serve as points of connection with others, even those we might be quick to dismiss as somehow different from ourselves.

Observe your impact. If your instinct for giving and kindness seems blocked, another tip is to get to know the people you want to help and take the time to witness how your help could impact them. This is especially true when giving to charity; research suggests that we derive more happiness from giving to charity when we know how the funds will be used to make a difference in the life of a particular recipient.[30] So it helps to seek out charities that offer this information, or to do your own research to understand the impact of your potential donation.

Find what motivates you. Although this chapter is about kindness as a well-being practice, that kind of thinking itself may reflect a Western bias. In one study, telling Americans that kindness was good for them made their acts of kindness even more beneficial to their well-being.[31] The same wasn't true of South Koreans. Nor did the South Koreans benefit from hearing how good kindness was for other people, perhaps because those benefits are obvious—or because that doesn't capture the kind of collective harmony that South Koreans care about. This just goes to show that there is more to learn about how to spread kindness across cultures and what motivates people to be kind.

A LIFE OF KINDNESS

When Aaron Harvey was arrested as a young man in 2014, facing over half a century in prison, he proved his innocence and was released 8 months later.

He sued the city of San Diego in federal court, citing civil rights violations, and won. He went on to study political science at UC Berkeley, pledging to help dismantle the law that put him in jail and to pursue a life where he could do acts of kindness for others, particularly those often marginalized in society.

Today, Harvey is a cofounder of Affect the Youth, an organization that provides scholarships, mentorships, and internships for underrepresented youth.

Harvey continues to follow his father's advice, being kind in his everyday life. In fact, Harvey is still in contact with Ronald, the man he bought Starbucks for and helped move into his new apartment. Thanks to Harvey's kindness, Ronald is now connected to resources.

Harvey chose kindness when life showed him otherwise. And through helping others thrive, he was able to thrive himself.

"You should never go 24 hours without doing something for someone who can't repay you," Harvey says. "There's going to be something that's going to come across you every day, if not multiple things, and you should lend a hand. And if you're not, you're not just doing that individual a disservice, but you're ultimately doing yourself a disservice, as well."

Chapter 3
Empathy

After 10 years serving in the Marines, Erik Ontiveros came home to his wife, a new baby, and life as a stay-at-home father. He was happy to be back, but he secretly was suffering.

His experiences during his three deployments to Iraq had led him to depression, post-traumatic stress disorder (PTSD), and substance abuse.

"Coming home, seeing my daughter for the first time, really brought a lot of guilt and shame of not feeling worthy of her," says Ontiveros. "I just didn't feel like I belonged or I was deserving."

For years, he stayed silent, pushing away friends and family who tried to help. When it got to be too much, he met with his social worker at the Veteran Affairs office and finally shared his truth.

"I had to surrender myself and that was hard, because the mentality of *you have to ask for help* or anything of that nature—[that means] you seem vulnerable or you were weak," says Ontiveros, "That would get you killed in combat."

Ontiveros talked about the psychological impact of warfare, the trauma and the nightmares, and the subsequent substance abuse. He talked about how he had kept it all secret, that he felt he now had a language barrier and was unable to communicate his feelings with those around him.

Ontiveros talked, and the case worker listened with an open and empathic ear. That opened a doorway for him to be able to talk with others from a place of vulnerability, especially fellow veterans he knew. And they, too, listened with empathy. It was healing.

"The real magic is having somebody who can listen and understand without judgment," says Ontiveros. "A lot of times that's what we're seeking: that when we talk to someone, they can actually listen. When you're able to sympathize or show actual true empathy, there's an ease and comfort. You're not alone."

THE BENEFITS OF EMPATHY

Empathy is our ability to resonate with the emotions of other people and imagine what they may be thinking and feeling. Because we all long to be understood, receiving empathy from someone (as Ontiveros did from his case worker) can be an important tool for healing from suffering or trauma.

But *receiving* empathy isn't the only way to benefit from it; it's also good for us when we *offer* empathy to others. Why? Because empathy fosters connection by helping us attend to people's needs, consider their mindset, and care about their well-being. And all of that can lead us to act with more compassion, creating stronger social bonds.

Those who study empathy differentiate between its two key elements: *affective empathy* (our ability to experience the emotions of others) and *cognitive empathy* (our ability to put ourselves in someone else's shoes and understand their thoughts).[1]

The two elements of empathy involve different parts of our brains that interact with each other in complex ways.[2] To experience emotional empathy, we rely on special cells in the brain called *mirror neurons* that fire when we see someone experience something we've experienced ourselves before (and help create a similar emotional reaction).[3] If we watch a scary movie and see the heroine walking toward obvious danger, we'll feel a bit nervous or scared too.

To experience cognitive empathy (imagining what another is thinking), we use our prefrontal cortex and temporal lobes—the parts of the brain that house our memories of past experiences and allow us to make inferences about someone else's mindset.[4, 5] For example, if someone is grieving a loss, we may understand they are not at their best and forgive any lapses in their manners or judgment.

As physician researcher Helen Riess writes in her book, *The Empathy Effect*,

> "[Your] sophisticated neurological system allows you to observe others hurting and gives you just enough of a taste of the pain to consider helping them out." This is important because "all parties are equally enriched when we perceive and respond to each other with empathy and compassion."[6]

EMPATHY DRIVES US TO HELP

Evidence of the ability to empathize has been seen in children as young as 8 months old through a child's visible reaction to their mother's distress.[7] Toddlers who see someone in need have the capacity to understand that that person's view of things may be different from their own, which allows them to potentially recognize another's pain or discomfort and step up to help.[8, 9]

Although the ability to empathize is not unique to humans, it's a skill that is highly evolved in humans, making altruistic action possible even under extraordinary circumstances.[10] Think of people who worked to hide Jewish people from Nazis during World War II—at great risk to themselves. No doubt, they were motivated by high levels of empathy, which is often tied to moral behavior and altruism.[11, 12] Empathy happens in much less extraordinary circumstances, too, leading to more kindness toward others and more cooperation in everyday life.[13]

EMPATHY MAKES YOU HAPPIER

Maybe you're asking yourself, is empathizing really good for our happiness?[14] The answer to that is a resounding yes. While it may not always feel great in the moment if we are resonating with people's uncomfortable feelings, the benefits are worth it because empathy shores up our relationships and our compassion, both key to happiness.[15]

"[I] see empathy and compassion as short-term costs in giving resources, whether it's time, energy, or emotional resources, to build stronger social relationships," says David DeSteno, a researcher who studies empathy. "I always recommend investing in other people, because the short-term cost is worth the long-term gain you'll get back in building strong relationships."

Along those lines, empathic people tend to attract friends and acquaintances through their ability to inspire trust in others.[16] Being empathic and showing emotional support to help those closest to us has been found to increase *our own* personal well-being in addition to that of those we're trying to help, probably because it makes us feel closer to the person in need.[17]

Our romantic relationships also improve when we approach them with empathy. In one study, 156 heterosexual couples from Pennsylvania and Massachusetts of different ages, ethnicities, and incomes—some married, some not—were videotaped while discussing difficult topics in their relationship.[18] Later, each member of the couple watched the videos and reported how they felt at different charged moments, how they thought their partner was feeling, and whether their partner was making an effort to empathize. Those who saw their partner trying to empathize with them felt much better about their relationship—even if their partner couldn't accurately read their emotions.

Empathy also has benefits at work. Empathic bosses can help create a healthy workforce, with employees experiencing reduced physical complaints like stomachaches or headaches and increased positive emotion, allowing them to be more productive.[19] The more empathic physicians are, according to their patients, the better the doctor/patient relationship, which also leads to better health for patients and less potential burnout for doctors.[20, 21, 22]

EMPATHY ACROSS OUR DIFFERENCES

Nurturing empathy can also help us get along better across different social groups. In one experiment, white and Asian undergraduates watched videotapes of a white person and a Black person going through experiences like shopping in a store or interacting with police—with the Black person experiencing poorer treatment—and were asked to either consider the viewpoint of the Black person or try to ignore his perspective and simply observe what happened.

Those students primed to empathize with the Black person expressed less subconscious bias toward Black people and interacted more warmly with a Black research assistant than those not instructed to empathize.[23] In fact, an analysis of several studies on prejudice found that increased empathy—specifically, the ability to take other people's perspectives—is one of the most important factors in bias reduction.[24]

Empathy can also lead to compassionate action across differences. In another study, participants listened to an interview with a heroin addict named Jared who'd been incarcerated for his crimes. Some participants were told to listen while keeping in mind how Jared was feeling and how his addiction affected his life, while others were told to listen impassively and take an objective position. Those who were asked to empathize with Jared reported feeling more sympathetic, compassionate, and tender toward him and were more inclined to allocate funds to a drug treatment center than the impassive group.[25]

Even though research is more often focused on empathy in hard situations, we can also resonate with people experiencing *positive* feelings—like the joy of getting engaged or the surprise of receiving a gift. When we share in people's delight, we *also* feel closer to them. Being able to feel happy for others matters for satisfying relationships and well-being too.[26]

As researcher Greg Depow found when studying everyday empathy, "Empathy is not always about engaging with the suffering of others. We also use it often to connect with other people's happiness, and that can be a way of feeling connected to those around us, too."

Of course, getting along with others isn't just important for our own well-being. It's also important for society as a whole. If we can understand how someone different from us might be feeling and thinking about their life situation, we are more apt to be able to see them as part of our circle of care. And that can build bridges and make us feel more united than divided.

Fortunately, our ability to empathize is not fixed, but can be built up over time by practicing it in different situations.[27] So, if you want to be happier yourself while building a better society through empathy, read on.

HOW EMPATHIC ARE YOU?

Before we offer you empathy practices to try out, we'd like to give you the opportunity to reflect on your own experiences of empathy.[28] If you'd like, you can revisit these questions later to see if taking steps to practice empathy made a difference.

	Strongly disagree	Disagree	Neutral	Agree	Strongly agree
When someone else is feeling excited, I tend to get excited too.	1	2	3	4	5
I sometimes find it difficult to see things from the other person's point of view.	5	4	3	2	1
I try to look at everybody's side of a disagreement before I make a decision.	1	2	3	4	5
I get a strong urge to help when I see someone who is upset.	1	2	3	4	5
I find that I am in tune with other people's moods.	1	2	3	4	5
I become irritated when someone cries.	5	4	3	2	1
I can easily imagine events that will make my friends happy.	1	2	3	4	5

	Strongly disagree	Disagree	Neutral	Agree	Strongly agree
I believe that there are at least two sides to every question and try to look at them all.	1	2	3	4	5
I enjoy making other people feel better.	1	2	3	4	5
Before criticizing somebody, I try to imagine how I would feel if I were in their place.	1	2	3	4	5

Quick scoring guide: 10–30 = Low; 31–40 = Medium; 41–50 = High

EMPATHY PRACTICES

PRACTICE #1: ACTIVE LISTENING

Time: 10 minutes

Read the steps of this practice, adapted from the book Fighting for Your Marriage, *and then plan out a time to try it.*

This listening practice can help your conversation partner feel more understood and help you feel more satisfied with your relationships.[29, 30]

Find a quiet place where you can talk with a conversation partner without interruption or distraction. Invite this person to share what's on their mind. As they do so, try to follow the steps below. You don't need to cover every step, but the more steps you follow, the more effective this practice is likely to be.

Paraphrase. Once the other person has finished expressing a thought, try to summarize what they said to make sure you understand and to show that you are paying attention. Helpful ways to paraphrase include "What I hear you saying is . . . ," "It sounds like . . . ," and "If I understand you right . . . ."

Ask questions. When appropriate, ask questions to encourage the other person to tell you more about their thoughts and feelings. Try to avoid jumping to conclusions about what the other person means. Instead, ask questions to clarify their meaning, such as, "When you say _____, do you mean _____?"

Express empathy. If the other person voices difficult feelings, try to validate these feelings rather than questioning or defending against them. If the speaker expresses frustration, try to consider why they feel that way. Respond with support and understanding, regardless of whether you think that feeling is justified or whether you would feel that way yourself if you were in their position. You might respond, "I can sense that you're feeling frustrated," or "I can understand how that situation could be frustrating."

Use engaged body language. You can show that you are engaged and interested by making eye contact, nodding, facing the other person, and maintaining an open and relaxed body posture. Try to avoid giving into distractions in your environment or checking your phone. Be mindful of your facial expressions, and avoid judgment. Your goal is to understand the other person's perspective and accept it for what it is, even if you disagree with it. Try not to interrupt with counterarguments or mentally prepare a rebuttal while the other person is speaking.

Avoid giving advice. If problem-solving is needed, it's likely to be more effective after people feel understood. Moving too quickly into advice giving may not be helpful.

It might feel awkward just to let someone talk when you probably have some thoughts to share. But many Science of Happiness students were pleasantly surprised to find that when they practiced Active Listening, their conversation partner appreciated it deeply—and often came up with solutions to their own problems, all on their own.

Take turns. After the other person has had a chance to speak and you have engaged in the active listening steps above, ask if it's okay for you to share your thoughts and feelings. When sharing your perspective, express yourself as clearly as possible using "I" statements (e.g., "I feel overwhelmed when you don't help out around the house"). It may also be helpful, when relevant, to express empathy for the other person's perspective (e.g., "I know you've been very busy lately and don't mean to leave me hanging").

Make a plan: List a few names of people you could try Active Listening with and ideas for when and where you could schedule it this week. Come back and write notes about how it went!

Who:
_____
_____

When:
_____
_____

How did it go? How did they respond to your interest?
Did you feel more connected?
_____
_____
_____
_____
_____

PUTTING EMPATHY INTO PRACTICE

If you're encountering other people during your day, you probably have many opportunities for empathy. In one study, on an average day, people had about nine opportunities to practice empathy—when other people expressed emotions in their presence—and six opportunities to receive empathy themselves.[31] That's why we say empathy is one of the building blocks of connection.

GETTING CURIOUS ABOUT OTHERS

Active Listening is one way to boost your empathy skills, and you may find it helpful to use those tips. Not only can it make other people feel heard and understood, but also it can help you learn things about them you may not have otherwise.

That's because we're not always as great at putting ourselves in other people's shoes as we think we are. Despite our best efforts, we can fall back on interpreting situations through our own biases and perspectives.[32] In most cases, it's better to ask someone what they feel or what they think rather than try to guess.

In addition to being curious in a conversation, another way to boost empathy is to be curious about the world and all the diverse experiences of people in it. Researcher Roman Krznaric suggests initiating conversations with people who don't necessarily share your interests and viewpoints—people from different political groups or religious persuasions, for example—and trying to engage strangers on the street.[33] When face-to-face interactions aren't possible, good alternatives are books, photographs, movies, and other art forms that help you imagine the interior lives of other people. If you're able to travel, that can also broaden your horizons.

"It helps to have a wide range of experiences yourself and some kind of knowledge of the kinds of lives that people live who are different from you," says researcher Heidi Maibom.[34]

AVOIDING DISTRESS AND OVERWHELM

At the end of the day, shoring up your empathy may be less about learning skills like Active Listening and more about staying motivated to empathize in situations when it's hard.[35]

"Our task is not to seek for empathy, but to search and find all the barriers that we built up against it," says GGSC science director Emiliana Simon-Thomas, one of the co-instructors of our Science of Happiness course, riffing off a quote from the poet Rumi.

So when do we turn off empathy, and how can we avoid doing that?

Being empathic for someone going through good times and sharing in their joy might come naturally. But the challenge might lie in empathizing with someone going through hard times—or, worse, someone blaming you for their pain or sorrow—when it could feel sad or uncomfortable to empathize.

Being in the presence of other people's pain and struggle can be hard to bear, especially if those people are close to us or if their struggles feel unsolvable, like the plight of refugees halfway across the world. It can be difficult to sustain our empathy and offer support if we feel overwhelmed ourselves by their suffering.

Research suggests that the first spark of empathy can evolve in one of two ways, either toward empathic distress or empathic concern.[36] Empathic concern is similar to compassion—it's a positive feeling that involves the desire to help. But empathic distress can lead to withdrawal, poor health, and burnout.

How can we stay present with other people's difficulty without getting overwhelmed ourselves? Here are some suggestions from the GGSC's Amy L. Eva:

- **Check in with yourself first.** What are you feeling, and what do you need in this moment? Take a deep breath and pause before you start to jump in and respond to someone.
- **Question your thoughts.** If a situation is particularly distressing you, you may be having other thoughts that are exacerbating your feelings. If a family member is calling you yet again for support, you

might imagine that they'll never be happy and independent. Questioning whether these thoughts are true, or finding another way to look at the situation—like seeing it as an opportunity to express your love, without expectations—can help.

- **Name the emotions you're feeling.** Communicate with someone who can support you, like a friend or therapist.[37]

Most importantly, we can try to shift away from empathic distress into empathic concern, or compassion. Simply helping or taking action is one way to alleviate distress, but you'll find many more compassion tips in the next chapter.

FINDING COMMON GROUND

Another barrier to empathy can arise not from the pain people are experiencing and how it makes us feel, but simply from who they are—and our own biases about them or their group.

We tend to empathize more easily with people we are emotionally closer to—our friends or family—than with strangers or people from social groups we're not affiliated with.[38] One study found that the parts of the brain that automatically resonate with others in pain are less active when we witness someone of a different race in pain compared to someone of our own race.[39] In addition, we're also less empathic to people when we believe they're responsible for their own suffering—for example, toward people who contracted HIV from drug use as opposed to a blood transfusion.[40] This has implications for how we feel about people living in poverty.

We also have trouble empathizing with someone who is farther away from us (distance-wise) than someone near us, which may explain why it can be harder to empathize with people across the world suffering hardship than with neighbors who live down the street.[41]

These biases aren't insurmountable. Studies have found that when we emphasize our commonality with others rather than our differences, we're more likely to empathize and be motivated to care.[42]

How can you find what you have in common with others? Try this practice:

PRACTICE #2: SHARED IDENTITY

Time: 10 minutes

This practice can help you expand the circle of your concern,[43] and it's often recommended in the context of healing our societal divisions.

1. **Choose a person in your life who seems to be very different from you in every way that you can imagine.** They might have different interests, different religious or political beliefs, or different life experiences. They might even be someone with whom you have had a personal conflict, or someone who belongs to a group that has been in conflict with one of your social groups.

You don't have to pick someone who makes you feel nervous or unsafe. If you've experienced inequities due to your race, sexuality, or gender, for example, you should not feel pressure to empathize with someone who has not shown you basic respect or decency.

Their name:
_____

2. **Make a list of the things that you most likely share in common with this person.** Perhaps you both work for the same company or go to the same school. Maybe you both have children or a significant other. Probably you have both had your heart broken at one point or another or have lost a loved one. Remind yourself that you and this person are both human beings.

Things we have in common:

_____

_____

_____

_____

_____

3. **Review the list you made.** Do the things you listed make you see this person in a new light? Instead of simply seeing this person as unfamiliar or as an outsider, try to see them as a human being, one whose tastes and experiences might overlap with yours in certain ways.
4. **Repeat this exercise.** Try it whenever you meet someone who initially seems different from you, has a conflict with you, or you feel uncomfortable around.

In the end, your beliefs about empathy matter. If you see empathy as something that can be learned, research finds that you'll be more likely to put in the effort to empathize in situations where to do so is challenging.[44] If you're like many of our Science of Happiness students, you just might be surprised how much other people appreciate it when you really tune into them.

When veteran Erik Ontiveros finally sought help for his PTSD, depression, and addictions, he found it through talking with his peers—his fellow veterans—who actively listened to him with empathy and nonjudgment.

After overcoming his own challenges, Ontiveros turned his attention to working with other veterans suffering from mental health issues, providing them with peer-to-peer support at Veterans Affairs clinics throughout rural, underserved communities in California.

Ontiveros wanted to further strengthen his listening skills with the veterans, so for our *Science of Happiness* podcast, he tried the Active Listening exercise during his Wednesday group counseling sessions.

It took some getting used to. He says it felt a bit robotic when he first tried it, especially the paraphrasing, where you make statements like, "What I hear you saying is . . ."

But after a little practice, Ontiveros not only got used to it, he thrived from it. The steps began to feel natural and authentic—especially the paraphrasing.

"Sometimes you may hear the person," Ontiveros says. "But you're not listening to what it is that they're trying to say. The paraphrasing allows you to do that. It shows that you are listening and really taking the time to understand."

Through Ontiveros's active listening, veterans opened up about their own struggles. One veteran in rehab shared his pain over not being able to be home with his family on his son's birthday.

Ontiveros easily could have given advice about how to move forward or how to talk to the son. "But that isn't my job," Ontiveros says. "My job is to validate this other veteran's thoughts and his feelings."

Instead of giving advice, Ontiveros used the Active Listening tool of asking for permission to share his own perspective. When he got a green light, he shared using "I" statements, like "Here's what I had to deal with," "Here's what my depression looks like," and "This is what I was able to do to help get myself out of that funk."

"I think 'I' statements are great," says Ontiveros. "When you give that perspective, you're giving your point of view as it's related to yourself. You share your own stories. Your own experiences."

In addition to using words, Ontiveros also relied on body language to convey his empathy through his posture, a smile, a nod, a hand gesture, or maintaining eye contact while someone spoke. He also learned to read other people's body language.

"Now I really take the time to listen and understand with all of my relationships," says Ontiveros. "When I can do that, it helps build the relationships—whether it be a friendship, a significant other, a family member, whoever, this is a great tool to make it stronger."

Chapter 4
Compassion

Contributing coauthor: Haley Gray

When rapper Rexx Life Raj created his album *The Blue Hour*, it was a way of processing the grief he was feeling. His mother had been taking care of his father, who had diabetes and heart failure, and then she was diagnosed with cancer herself. Raj became her caregiver, and he tried to handle everything on his own, sharing with few people in his life about what was going on. Then in 2021, both of his parents passed away within 4 months of each other.

All the pain of that time went into his album, alongside the world's collective isolation and loss around the pandemic. One of the songs went:

> *Tellin' me that it's ok*
> *Sounds just like lies*
> *How am I supposed to live without you*
> *I'll try...*
> *All of it was hard*
> *So why is it so hard to cry?*
> *All the weight I've lifted*
> *Ain't heavy as this heart of mine*

Raw and real, his music became a source of support to fans who were also grieving. On tour in Ohio, he met one of those fans, a man whose mother had stage 4 cancer.

"We talked for a second, but I could see like he really wanted to cry," recalls Raj. "He was trying to hold it in and he was trying to be strong."

In that moment, Raj saw a mirror of his own pain and his own struggles to stay tough while "dying inside."

"I remember telling him . . . you don't have to hold it in, bro. What you're going through, it's hard to wrap your mind around it; you don't have to be strong in this moment," Raj says.

The man cried, and the two cried together—a moment of compassion. Having gone through a similar experience himself, Raj was able to be a witness to his fan's suffering, and to make space for him to let down his defenses.

Later, Raj cried backstage as he realized what his music meant to people. "What I want[ed] is just a place where people could come and we could hold a space for these feelings and these emotions," he says. "It really dawned on me like, man, you put what you went through into this music and it's connecting with people."

> **WHAT ARE THE DIFFERENCES BETWEEN COMPASSION, EMPATHY, AND KINDNESS?**
>
> Many people confuse compassion with empathy or kindness—even researchers, at times. But, while empathy is often a precursor[1] to compassion because resonating with others' emotions helps us understand they're in need, and kindness can be compassion's natural outcome, compassion is distinct from both of these, involving its own neural networks and different practices for enhancing it.
>
> Let's say you see a person living on the street and you imagine they're hurting and sad, watching indifferent people walk by every day. You may resonate with their pain (i.e., feel empathy), which

> could attune you to their suffering. But, unless you feel compassion, you are less likely to stop and take action to help them (i.e., show kindness).

THE BENEFITS OF COMPASSION

The essence of compassion is a warm feeling of caring concern coupled with the motivation to ease suffering—and it's a natural instinct that can be nurtured with deliberate practice.[2] Compassion is good for our well-being, as well as for other people's well-being. That makes compassion yet another important key to happiness.

The deep biological basis for compassion starts with parent–child bonding.[3] When we care about the well-being of our children, hormones like oxytocin are released into our bloodstream, which have effects on our physiology and feelings. Oxytocin can help slow down our heart rate, and it stimulates the parts of our brains connected to empathy, caregiving, and pleasure.[4,5] Perhaps that's why research has found that parents trained to be compassionate can effectively reduce stress not only in themselves but in their children too.[6]

When we feel compassion, we experience changes in brain activity that may lead to kind behavior. In one study, participants in Wisconsin who completed a 2-week daily training in compassion showed increased activity in areas of their brains associated with empathy, planning, emotional control, and reward in comparison to other participants who trained in reframing emotions. These neural changes led the compassion trainees to be more generous toward someone they witnessed being treated unfairly in a game.[7]

Compassion can be good for our relationships, helping build trust and love between people. Research suggests that compassionate people are considered particularly attractive as potential mates and make good friends.[8] At work, colleagues who show compassionate care for one another help create a closer, more efficient, and more productive work team.[9] And, as many spiritual and philosophical traditions have argued, compassion is important for fostering morality and preventing societal decay, making it a necessity for safe and happy communities.

Theologian and activist Desmond Tutu said, "We are each made for goodness, love, and compassion. We are transformed as much as the world is when we live with these truths." By caring about others' suffering and taking steps to alleviate it, we help create an environment of mutual care that benefits all of us. For that reason alone, it's important to nurture our compassionate instinct. But there are other reasons, too—including how compassion increases our own well-being.

COMPASSION MAKES US HAPPIER

The Dalai Lama said, "If you want others to be happy, practice compassion. If you want to be happy, practice compassion"—and scientific research backs up his philosophy.

In one study, researchers showed videos of people in distress to young women in Europe before and after training some of them in a compassion practice called *Metta* meditation, from the Buddhist tradition. This practice involves wishing others well—starting with someone you love, then people farther and farther from your intimate circle until you are embracing the whole world with your care. It's similar to the Compassion Meditation later in this chapter.

By using fMRI technology as people watched the videos, the researchers found that participants trained in compassion experienced more activity in brain regions associated with positive feelings and affiliation with others—compared to the control group trained in memory retention—even when witnessing people in distress.[10]

Study coauthor Olga Klimecki of the Max Planck Institute says that this finding suggests compassion training helps prevent people from being overwhelmed by others' suffering, leaving them better able to cope and respond in kind and helpful ways.

"When we share the suffering of others too much, our negative emotions increase. It carries the danger of an emotional burnout." But, she adds, "Through compassion training, we can increase our resilience and approach stressful situations with more positive [emotion]."

Research has found that cultivating compassionate feelings can decrease depression and make us feel more satisfied with life, mindful, and happy.[11] For adults with recurrent symptoms of depression and anxiety, training in compassion can improve symptoms, leading to reduced unpleasant feelings and increased positive feelings for up to 3 months, compared to people waiting for the training.[12]

Compassion can even help victims of trauma. In one study, veterans suffering from PTSD were offered one of two programs—a compassion-focused meditation or an educational course about PTSD and how to relax and sleep better. Those who did the compassion training had greater decreases in PTSD symptoms than those in the other group.[13] Similarly, a meditation course emphasizing how to cultivate compassion was offered to American women victims of violence who were suffering severe mental health issues. They had more improvements in their mental health and had reduced trauma symptoms compared to a control group who received normal trauma care without compassion meditation.[14]

COMPASSION MAKES US HEALTHIER

The benefits of compassion also extend to our physical health. People who feel more compassion have better heart rate variability, which tends to go along with soothing feelings and less overreacting to potentially threatening situations.[15] That means compassion likely helps us manage stressful situations better in the moment.

This held true in one study in San Francisco, where more compassionate women doing a stressful task (an impromptu speech that was evaluated by observers) had better physiological responses after the activity, including lower blood pressure, lower cortisol spikes, and higher heart rate variability. The more compassionate folks seemed to make better use of social supports available to them, too, suggesting that compassion can be an important ingredient in good relationships.[16]

Findings like these may explain why compassion seems to help people facing difficult medical diagnoses. In one study, people with HIV completed questionnaires and interviews every six months for 17 years to see if giving or receiving compassionate love made a difference in their well-being. The researchers found that those who showed more compassion toward others had better survival rates, even when considering substance use and social support that may have affected their longevity too.[17]

In general, practicing compassion helps us cope with the ups and downs of life and also be better prepared to respond to others in need. It both *does* good and (generally) *feels* good at the same time. To learn more about how you can nurture compassionate feelings in your own life, read on.

HOW COMPASSIONATE ARE YOU?

Before we offer you compassion practices to try out, we'd like to give you the opportunity to reflect on your own experiences of compassion.[18] If you'd like, you can revisit these questions later to see if taking steps to practice compassion made a difference.

	Strongly disagree	Disagree	Neutral	Agree	Strongly agree
I pay careful attention when other people talk to me about their troubles.	1	2	3	4	5
If I see someone going through a difficult time, I try to be caring toward that person.	1	2	3	4	5
I am unconcerned with other people's problems.	5	4	3	2	1

I notice when people are upset, even if they don't say anything.	1	2	3	4	5
I like to be there for others in times of difficulty.	1	2	3	4	5
I think little about the concerns of others.	5	4	3	2	1
My heart goes out to people who are unhappy.	1	2	3	4	5
I try to avoid people who are experiencing a lot of pain.	5	4	3	2	1
When others feel sadness, I try to comfort them.	1	2	3	4	5
I can't really connect with other people when they're suffering.	5	4	3	2	1

Quick scoring guide: 10–30 = Low; 31–40 = Medium; 41–50 = High

COMPASSION PRACTICES

PRACTICE #1: COMPASSION MEDITATION

Time: 10 to 30 minutes

Research suggests that engaging in compassion meditation for 2 weeks can increase your generosity and lead to brain changes associated with compassion.[19] Longer mindfulness and compassion programs that include these meditations can help improve well-being and reduce distress and reactivity to stress.[20, 21, 22]

There are many versions of compassion meditation available online. We invite you to listen to the one at ggia.berkeley.edu/practice/compassion_meditation from researcher Helen Weng and her colleagues at the Center for Healthy Minds, which has seven steps, moving from easier forms of compassion to ones that may be harder:

- **Settling:** Get into a comfortable position and begin by focusing on your breath, noticing the sensations of breathing.
- **Loving-kindness and compassion for a loved one:** Picture someone who is close to you, someone toward whom you feel a great amount of love. Notice how this love feels in your heart. Notice the sensations around your heart. Perhaps you feel a sensation of warmth, openness, and tenderness. Continue breathing, and focus on these feelings as you visualize your loved one. As you breathe out, imagine that you are extending a golden light that holds your warm feelings from the center of your heart. Imagine that the golden light reaches out to your loved one, bringing them peace and happiness. At the same time, silently recite these phrases:
  - May you be free from suffering.
  - May you have joy and happiness.
  - May you experience joy and ease.
- **Compassion for a loved one:** Repeat the previous step, but for a loved one who is suffering. Notice how you feel when you think of their suffering. Do the sensations change?
- **Compassion for self:** Repeat the previous step, but for yourself, remembering a time when you suffered.
- **Compassion for a neutral person:** Repeat the previous step, but for someone you neither like nor dislike—someone you may see in your everyday life, such as a classmate you don't know, a bus driver, or a stranger you pass on the street—keeping in mind how they might have suffered in their life.
- **Compassion for an enemy:** Repeat the previous step, but for someone with whom you have difficulty in your life—a parent or child you disagree with, an ex, a roommate you had an argument with, or a coworker you don't get along with—keeping in mind how they have suffered in their life.
- **Compassion for all beings:** End with a wish for all other beings' suffering to be relieved. Just as we wish to be peaceful, happy, and free from suffering, so do all beings. Bask in the joy of this openhearted wish to ease

the suffering of all people and how this attempt might bring joy, happiness, and compassion in your heart at this very moment.

REFLECT

Write freely about your experience with this Compassion Meditation. Did you notice any sensations or reactions? When would you like to practice it again?

PRACTICE #2: FEELING SUPPORTED

Time: 15 minutes

Research suggests that this practice can help foster your compassion by guiding you to recall times others have comforted you.[23]

1. Make a list of the people who offer you comfort or security. If it's helpful, consider:
   – Who is the person you most like to spend time with?
   – Who is the person it is hardest to be away from?
   – Who is the person you want to talk to when you are worried about something?

– Who is the person you turn to when you are feeling down?
– Who is the person you know will always be there for you?
– Who is the person you want to share your successes with? (Some of these might be the same person.)

2. Write down six positive qualities that are common to some or all of these people—qualities that they strongly demonstrate.

3. Next, recall and visualize a specific situation when you were feeling distressed or worried, and one of these people comforted and helped you.
4. Write a brief description of that situation and the way you felt during it.

PUTTING COMPASSION INTO PRACTICE

Compassion is a feeling, but when we think about expressing our compassion, we typically imagine offering heartfelt words or actually helping someone in need.

But there is a wide range of ways to be compassionate. For example, touch is a powerful way to show your compassion without even the need for words.

In one study, researchers asked young adults in California (mainly white, Chinese, or Korean) to try to communicate a dozen emotions with a 1-second touch on someone's arm through a barrier, so the person couldn't see them. Remarkably, people receiving the touch were able to identify compassion nearly 60% of the time.[24]

"A pat on the back, a caress of the arm—these are everyday, incidental gestures that we usually take for granted, thanks to our amazingly dexterous hands.... They are our primary language of compassion, and a primary means for spreading compassion," writes Dacher Keltner, a coauthor of the study and co-instructor of our Science of Happiness course.

On the other hand, sometimes compassion looks much less warm and fuzzy than we might imagine—it manifests as *tough* compassion. This might involve taking a stand and making uncomfortable choices for the greater good.

"If your aunt makes an offhand racist remark, or your work buddy insults a colleague, tough compassion involves speaking up—without rancor, but with conviction—if your goal is to promote less suffering for all," writes author Elizabeth Svoboda.[25]

So how do we boost our compassion, in all its forms? If we want to feel concern for the suffering of others, we first have to notice it.[26] "It is hard to sometimes see when people need help, especially if we're not looking for it," says one Science of Happiness student, Kit John from Cleveland, Ohio.

To start, psychologist Rick Hanson suggests that we tune in to the faces of those around us:

> *Watch and listen to those closest to you. What's hurting over there? Face it, even if you have to admit that you are one of its causes. If appropriate, ask some questions, and talk about the answers. . . . Look at faces—at work, walking down the street, in the mall, across the dinner table. Notice the weariness, the bracing against life, the wariness, irritability, and tension. Sense the suffering behind the words.*[27]

Suffering isn't always so obvious. Sometimes, it can come out as—or be masked by—defensiveness or aggression. "If someone, even a loved one, confronts me with anything that seems unduly critical or confrontational . . . they are usually doing so because they feel insecure and vulnerable," says Science of Happiness student Jacob Shin from New York. Sometimes, a compassionate response that speaks to their potential underlying hurt can defuse any surface anger. That might be as simple as asking someone how their workday was, if they seem unusually short or snippy with you right after they arrive home. Compassion, in this scenario, involves giving them the benefit of the doubt.

Just as with empathy, we may be more compassionate toward people who are more similar to us than different, live close to us, or share our beliefs. If you find yourself unmoved by the suffering of a certain person or group, again, you can try to imagine what you have in common with them rather than focusing on your differences.

As you work on building compassion, Santa Clara University professor

Hooria Jazaieri suggests noticing moments during the day when you feel compassionate or, on the flip side, when you avoid being compassionate.[28] Notice when you embraced your crying child or spoke to someone experiencing homelessness in your community. When relevant, you can also notice how good it felt to show your compassion—to be warm, loving, and wishing well for others.

AVOIDING COMPASSION FATIGUE

You might remember that, in the previous chapter, we suggested compassion as an antidote to feelings of distress that can arise when we face overwhelming emotions in others. And while that's true, even our compassion can break down when we're repeatedly exposed to suffering and need—especially suffering we cannot alleviate. This state of burnout and overwhelm, called compassion fatigue, was originally identified in the health care industry and includes a breakdown in compassion, alongside other physical and mental health symptoms.

The antidotes are much the same—namely, to take care of yourself and to identify concrete ways you can help. If necessary, says researcher Daryl Cameron, settle on ways to help that are less costly to you.[29] Perhaps you can't drive someone to all their medical appointments, but you can check in with them on the phone afterward.

"Once you've decided what kind of response is consistent with your values, commit to taking some sort of concrete action—however humble . . . whether it's starting a website, donating to a local charity, or booking a volunteer shift," writes Svoboda.[30]

One thing that should help you sustain your compassion in the long run is feeling your actions make a difference, seeing yourself as "very good at responding compassionately to those in trouble."[31] Interestingly, people who have gone through adversity in the past have an increased sense of efficacy in dealing with others' suffering in the present.[32] If you are confronted with suffering, connecting it to your own struggles might help.

If the plight of refugees around the world feels insurmountable, you could remember your own overwhelming experience of moving to a new city. With that in mind, you might think about donating books and clothes to a refugee center, or making sure to help someone who seems lost navigating public transit.

Svoboda also recommends joining a community of helpers.[33] That way, your compassionate action is no longer a drop in the bucket but part of a larger movement, making it feel more impactful.

None of this means compassion is easy. Those of us caring day in and day out for people who are suffering know how hard it can be. Especially when there is little we can do, what remains for us is to simply be mindful of and present with their pain, to the best of our ability, without feeling we have to make it go away. And to forgive ourselves when even that feels too difficult.

Here, again, Hanson's words may help:

> *Let the pain of the other person wash through you. Don't resist it. Opening your heart, finding compassion—the sincere wish that a being not suffer—will lift and fuel you to bear the other's pain. We long to feel received by others; turn it around: Your openness to another person, your willingness to be moved, is one of the greatest gifts you can offer.*
>
> *To sustain this openness, it helps to have a sense of your own body. Tune into breathing, and steady the sense of being here with the other person's issues and distress over there.*
>
> *Have heart for yourself as well. It's often hard to bear the pain of others, especially if you feel helpless to do anything about it. It's okay if your response is not perfect.*[34]

When Raj did the Compassion Meditation for our *Science of Happiness* podcast, he imagined a family member—someone who was going through a lot at the time and had also been through a lot as a child. But she was a little difficult to be compassionate toward, since she had a temper and sometimes rubbed people the wrong way.

Through the meditation, Raj came to see that her behavior was understandable, that she was doing her best, and that he wanted the best for her. Afterward, he sent her a text message to check how she was doing.

She was appreciative, and they ended up chatting back and forth about their lives.

"[The practice] put me in the headspace to even reach out," says Raj. "'Cause without the meditation, I probably wouldn't even have."

For Raj, a simple check-in like that was the kind of support he had wanted and needed when he was dealing with his parents' illnesses and deaths.

"That was a big thing when going through grief. . . . It's not even that I wanted people to say certain things to me, but I wanted it to be known that you were thinking about me," he says.

Sometimes, being compassionate isn't all that complicated. It just takes our time and presence. Raj says, "I just wanted to let her know, even though we don't talk all the time, I'm here if you ever need anything and I'm thinking of you."

Chapter 5
Awe

When musician Diana Gameros arrived in Mexico, she felt disconnected from her surroundings, almost as if in a dream.

Sixteen years had passed since Gameros was last in her home country. As a teenager, she said goodbye to her family and moved to Michigan from Juárez.

"There's this thing that I believe immigrants have to do when we're away from our homeland," says Gameros. "Which is to block this emotional connection that we have to our land in order for us to cope."

But Gameros wanted to feel connected—to savor every single moment she was there. So for our *Science of Happiness* podcast, she chose to do an Awe Outing practice at the Zócalo, Mexico City's bustling main city square.

For the Awe Outing, you shift your awareness so that you are open to what is around you, to things that are vast, impressively complex, or surprising and delightful. So Gameros turned off her phone and began focusing on her breathing and the sights and sounds around her.

She took in the beauty of the colonial buildings and majestic cathedrals surrounding the square. She watched vendors selling an array of goods, people walking alone, couples holding hands and whispering to one another, children laughing, and the distant sounds of someone playing a street organ.

"The Zócalo is a very powerful place," says Gameros. "It's very big and colorful. There are so many sounds and people, and so much history. My senses were opened. I connected through my walk, by slowing down and then shifting my awareness to what was around me. I had been there for about a month and somehow I couldn't believe it. I couldn't feel it—until I did this practice. Then I finally felt present in Mexico."

THE BENEFITS OF AWE

When we are in the presence of something extraordinary or vast, like Mexico City's Zócalo, it can fill us with a sense of wonder and challenge our understanding of the world and our place in it. That experience of feeling small in the presence of something greater than ourselves is what researchers call awe. It, too, is a key to happiness.

We can feel awe in many circumstances, including when we witness a spectacular sunset, a baby being born, or an extremely generous or courageous act. We can experience awe alone, when hiking solo in an ancient redwood forest, or with others, when watching extraordinary athletic feats in a crowded sports arena. And it can come upon us spontaneously or be cultivated purposefully by tuning into our senses and paying closer attention to the amazing world around us—such as noticing the complexity of a single flower or, as our *Science of Happiness* podcast guest found, attending to a city's special beauty.

AWE, YOUR BODY, AND YOUR RELATIONSHIPS

Scientists have found that awe is a unique emotion that has its own signature effects on our bodies and brains.[1] Experiencing awe decreases activity in our sympathetic nervous system, which is tied to our fight-or-flight response, and goes along with stronger vagal tone—meaning, our calming, parasympathetic nervous system is working better with our hearts.[2] What this all means for us is that feeling awe equips us to handle stress and also recover, preparing us to attend to the people around us with calm and care.

Experiencing awe when witnessing moral, courageous acts can stimulate the release of oxytocin—sometimes called the *tend and befriend* hormone, because its release encourages trust and care for others.[3] Feeling awe also coincides with decreased activation in the default network of our brains, making us less self-focused and ruminative.

Thanks to the wonder and calm we feel, and the reduced self-focus, awe encourages us to be kinder and more generous—even in children as young as 8 years old.[4, 5] In experiments where young adults recalled awe experiences, looked at beautiful nature videos, or simply looked up in a grove of tall eucalyptus trees, they were more likely to help someone in need and less likely to feel entitled or act unethically than those who were not feeling awe.[6]

In fact, awe has been found to make us feel more globally connected to others and more willing to act generously toward people far away from us.[7] As researcher Sean Laurent explains, "When you get people thinking in these ways—like I'm just one grain of sand among all of the other grains of sand on the beach—it actually leads to a more cosmopolitan prosociality, where you want to help people who are further away."

This was reflected in Jools Morgan-Jones's experience practicing awe through our Science of Happiness course. "Awe has humbled me, delighted me, and made me consider my place in the world," she says. "It has made me more inclined to realize the interconnectedness of things and creatures on this spinning ball of green and blue, and to prompt me to reach out to help my fellow creatures, human or otherwise."

AWE HELPS OUR MENTAL AND PHYSICAL HEALTH

Research also finds that feeling awe increases our well-being. In one study across the United States and Spain, the more awe people felt on a daily basis, the less stressed and more satisfied with life they felt, above and beyond the effects of other positive emotions, like amusement and joy.[8] Awe seems to keep us focused on the present—whatever we are experiencing in the moment—which makes time feel as if it has slowed down.[9] This leads to better decision making, more patience with others, and simply more enjoyment of life.

Experiencing awe affects happiness in other ways too. For one, when we feel awe, we tend to simultaneously experience other positive emotions—such as compassion, gratitude, love, and optimism—as well as a stronger sense of connectedness with others.[10]

"When I am in awe, I am also very grateful for the miracle of life," says Science of Happiness student Bertha Rosa Camacho from Switzerland.

At the same time, awe seems to help us handle sour moods. Several studies have found that walking in nature rather than urban settings makes us feel calmer, show fewer unpleasant emotions and stress, and ruminate less—rumination being a telltale feature of depression.[11] This has led to a whole body of research looking at the ways that being in nature can improve our mood and well-being, in some cases leading to calls for increased access to nature at a societal level.[12] Though the reasons nature is good for us are many, at least some studies find that its benefits are partially due to the feelings of awe it inspires.[13]

Awe isn't just helpful for increasing well-being in people who are already thriving, though. It can also help those experiencing extreme hardship. In one study, veterans with PTSD and youth from impoverished neighborhoods were taken on guided river rafting trips in California or Utah to help them have an immersive experience in nature.[14] According to analyses of their journals and surveys, participants who experienced more awe had increases in their overall well-being and fewer stress-related symptoms after the trip was over.

Awe can have benefits not just for our emotional health, but for our physical health, too.[15] When researchers in the United States looked at people's daily lives during the COVID-19 pandemic, they found that people feeling more awe experienced less stress, better sleep, and fewer headaches.[16] Awe has also been found to affect our immune system directly. In one study, young adults experiencing awe regularly had lower levels of interleukin-6—a cytokine (small protein) tied to inflammation—while experiencing other positive emotions such as joy or contentment didn't have this effect.[17]

As awe researcher Dacher Keltner says of this study, "That awe, wonder, and beauty promote healthier levels of cytokines suggests that the things we do to experience these emotions—a walk in nature, losing oneself in music, beholding art—have a direct influence upon health and life expectancy."

For all of these reasons, awe is an important emotion to experience in everyday life. However, we must keep in mind that awe can be triggered not only by wonderful things, but also by fearful or troubling events—for example, wild, dangerous thunderstorms or being in a large group listening to a speech by a charismatic despot. This *negative awe* doesn't produce the same neural activity as positive awe and may not have the same corresponding health benefits.[18, 19]

Fortunately, the vast majority of awe experiences people have in everyday life *are* positive, and positive awe experiences are pretty easy to access just by getting a small dose of nature.[20] If you want to find out other ways to cultivate positive awe in your life, read on.

ARE YOU PRONE TO EXPERIENCING AWE?

Before we offer you awe practices to try out, we'd like to give you the opportunity to reflect on your own experiences of awe.[21] If you'd like, you can revisit these questions later to see if taking steps to cultivate awe made a difference.

	Strongly disagree	Disagree	Neutral	Agree	Strongly agree
I often feel childlike wonder in the face of new experiences, ideas, or scenes of nature.	1	2	3	4	5
When I see someone do something incredible, I feel tingles down my spine or get goose bumps.	1	2	3	4	5

I feel a positive, emotional connection to nature.	1	2	3	4	5
I seek out experiences that challenge my understanding or expectations about the world.	1	2	3	4	5
It's hard for me to think of anyone who really impresses or inspires me.	5	4	3	2	1
I am rarely surprised or moved by things I see or experience in life.	5	4	3	2	1
I take many opportunities to explore the beauty of nature.	1	2	3	4	5
When people say "Wow" about a vista or sunset, I just don't get it.	5	4	3	2	1
I get caught up in the wonderment of life.	1	2	3	4	5
I avoid experiences that are unpredictable or out of my comfort zone.	5	4	3	2	1

Quick scoring guide: 10–30 = Low; 31–40 = Medium; 41–50 = High

AWE PRACTICES

PRACTICE #1: AWE OUTING

Time: 15 minutes

Read the steps of this practice now, and then plan out a time to try it.

This practice is designed to help you turn an ordinary outing into a series of awe-inspiring moments filled with delightful surprises, and research suggests it can help you feel more joyful, appreciative, and compassionate.[22]

To get started, turn off your phone. Phones and other devices can be distracting and draw your attention away from what's happening around you. Even better, don't bring your phone with you at all so that you won't be tempted to check it. Then, set off on your outing to a place of your choosing. (See below for ideas.)

During your outing, try to approach what you see, hear, smell, or otherwise sense with fresh eyes, imagining that you're experiencing it for the first time. Then, follow these steps:

1. Take a deep breath in. Count to six as you inhale and seven as you exhale. Feel the air move through your nose and hear the sound of your breath. Come back to this breath throughout your outing.
2. As you get going, feel the ground beneath you and the air on your skin, listen to surrounding sounds, and smell what is wafting around nearby.
3. Shift your awareness so that you are open to what is around you, to things that are vast, impressively complex, unexpected, or unexplainable, or that surprise and delight you.
4. Take another deep breath in. Again, count to six as you inhale and seven as you exhale.
5. Let your attention be open in exploration for what inspires awe. Is it a wide landscape? The tiny patterns of light and shadow? An

appliance or piece of furniture? Let your attention move from the vast to the small.

6. Ask yourself far-fetched questions: What is new, unknown, or unexplored about what is around you?

7. Continue your outing and, every so often, bring your attention back to your breath. Count to six as you inhale and seven as you exhale. Notice—really notice—the many sights, sounds, smells, and other sensations that are dancing through your awareness, usually undetected.

High school teacher Aran Levasseur took his students on an Awe Outing among the forests and hills of their beautiful school campus, and he was in awe of the profound experiences they had. One student said, "Seeing the way the water trickled and the way the light fractured and rippled on the rocks underneath amazed me. It felt like looking at art." Another reflected:

> *The way the branches of another plant latch on to the tree shows how interconnected each living thing is and how we might help or harm one another. This scene makes me wonder: What am I connected to? What might I help or harm? These questions provoke a sense of wonder and curiosity about relationships.*

Levasseur found the Awe Outings offered his students a respite from the competitive pressure of high school. "These walks were meaningful because they allowed us to slow down, reflect, enjoy the moment, and refocus and reset," he writes.[23]

Once you get in the habit of taking outings like this, you may be surprised by how often you have opportunities to experience awe—they are practically infinite.

> "There is a calming force among the tangle of trees in the absence of straight lines and corners. The moment of awe arrives unannounced when there are no words for the beauty you behold. Breathe it in and let it out." —**Science of Happiness student Mark M.**

As you move through your day, take note of the moments that bring you wonder, that give you goose bumps or make your chest feel broader: These are your opportunities for awe. They may be found in your neighborhood, in front of art, while listening to music, or while doing something together with other people.

Here are some specific ideas for Awe Outing destinations.

Natural settings:
- A local park or garden
- A mountain or hilltop with panoramic views
- A trail lined with tall trees
- The shore of an ocean, lake, river, or waterfall
- A clear night when you can see the stars
- A place where you can watch a sunset or sunrise

Urban settings:
- A yard, low-traffic sidewalk, or school playground
- The top of a skyscraper . . . or looking up in an area dense with tall buildings
- A historic monument
- A part of your city that you've never explored before
- A large ballpark or stadium
- Botanical gardens or a zoo with plants and animal species you've never seen before
- No destination; see where the outing takes you

Indoor settings:
- A library
- A gallery or hallway with art on the walls
- A planetarium or aquarium
- A historic mansion, cathedral, or opera house
- A museum

Make a plan: List a few easy-to-access places where you could try an Awe Outing, as well as a plan for the days and times that you could do it this week. Come back and journal about how it went!

My Awe Outing plan:

How did it go? How did you feel, and what drew your attention?

PRACTICE #2: NOTICING NATURE

Time: 10 minutes

Read the steps of this practice, based on research by Holli-Anne Passmore, and then plan out a time to try it.

This practice helps you turn your attention to the nature you encounter in everyday life, and research suggests it can help you cultivate positive emotions, a sense of connectedness, and kindness.[24]

1. **Be mindful of nature.** Give special attention to the natural elements and objects around you on a daily basis (e.g., trees, clouds, leaves, the moon, moving water, and animals). Ask yourself and notice: How do these make you feel? What emotions do they bring up? Take a moment to allow yourself to fully experience the nature around you.

2. **Take a photo.** When you encounter a natural object or scene that evokes a strong emotion in you, that moves you in some way, take a photo of it. You can use any type of camera that's available to you. Don't worry too much about the quality of the photo or how creative it is. Remember that tuning in to what you are photographing is more important.

3. **Describe your photo.** Write a short description of why you took the photo and how the nature scene made you feel. This can be a few words or a few sentences. If you'd like, share your photo with others or even have it printed.

4. **Repeat.** You can take as many photos as you like, but try to take at least 10 photos over the course of two weeks. You might even aim to take one photo each day. Be mindful of how the nature you encounter makes you feel on a daily basis.

Make a plan: List a few easy-to-access places where you could Notice Nature (e.g., a local park, a sidewalk at sunset) and a plan for the days and times that you could do it this week. Come back and write about how it went!

My Noticing Nature plan:

How did it go? What did you notice that felt new or inspired your curiosity?

PUTTING AWE INTO PRACTICE

According to one study, young adults in the United States tend to experience awe at least two times a week.[25]

Where do you find awe, and how can you seek out more of it? Keltner and his colleagues surveyed participants from 26 countries, speaking 20 different languages, on their stories of awe. The researchers distilled the answers into the eight most common sources of awe, which might help inspire your awe seeking[26]:

Moral beauty. Seeing courage, kindness, strength, or resilience in others can give us a sense of wonder, whether it's the heroic activism of former South African president Nelson Mandela or the earnest generosity of our own children.

Collective effervescence. It's *awe*some when we feel merged with others in a collective. This might happen at a wedding or graduation, a sporting event, or a political rally.

Nature. While moral beauty is actually the most common source of awe,[27] for many of us, awe and nature go hand in hand. Big natural events like eclipses, the vast night sky, and the majesty of mountains and oceans can make us go "wow."

Music. Vocal and instrumental music, from rock bands to religious chants, can profoundly move us. Science of Happiness student Leanne Hunt from South Africa, who is visually impaired, often finds awe in music:

> *. . . a large orchestra, a choir, a lone folk singer, a trio of violinists, or a band playing in a church. The sensation is one of inner swelling, like an expansion of my chest and a feeling of lightness, as if I may be lifted up from the ground.*

Art and visual design. Human creations, from buildings and pyramids to graffiti and paintings, can thrill our eyes and minds. As Science of Happiness student Kelli Karg says,

> *From innovations I've seen in Singapore to old forts, circles, churches, civilizations, I get chills and feel dumbstruck, but it almost always promotes my desire to learn MORE about that building, that group of people who made such things come to be.*

Spirituality and religion. Awe arises when we are in the presence of something vast or extraordinary, so it's no wonder that experiences of the sacred, transcendent, or divine often fill our hearts with awe.

Encountering life and death. Witnessing beings enter and leave this world is profound. "When I first saw my son, I experienced that awe moment. It was unbelievable to give birth to a perfect new baby and I am the creator," recalls Science of Happiness student Swati Smita, PhD, from India. "No experience matched with that moment of wonder, enchantment, and awe!"

Big ideas or epiphanies. Our minds expand when we are struck with philosophical insights, marvel at scientific discoveries, or realize things about ourselves—like the vastness of space or the miraculous workings of the human heart.

While these sources of awe are common across cultures, there are still cultural differences in how we experience awe. In studies with American and Chinese participants, researchers found that Americans tend to experience more awe from their own accomplishments, more awe from nature and architecture, and more positive versions of awe than Chinese people do. On the other hand, Chinese people tend to experience more awe in response to other people, and more fearful awe.[28] The physical experience of awe may be different, too, tending to be more calming in the United States and more activating in China.[29, 30]

While our commonalities reveal something about the human experience of awe, further research on awe across cultures will provide a more comprehensive picture of all its variations.

TIPS FOR CULTIVATING AWE

With all these different sources of awe, there are opportunities to experience it all around us. It just takes a little awareness and intention to see the world with fresh eyes. Here are some tips for opening your mind to awe:

Slow down. We can find awe in the everyday if we make a little space for it amid our busy lives. Science of Happiness student Leslie Sheridan from California looks for awe that's hiding in plain sight—"a tiny flower emerging between two sidewalk cracks, or a beautiful potted plant on someone's stoop, or the broad smile of a person on the street." She says, "In a world filled with so much beauty and inspiration, it's fairly easy to find awe in the course of a day . . . especially if one has 'open eyes' with which to see it."

Appreciate your senses. Awe can be a full sensory experience of color, texture, scent, and sound.

Researchers Michael Amster and Jake Eagle suggest seeking out awe as you cook, in the smells of ingredients, the heat of the oven, and your own movements. You can also find everyday awe while bathing, they point out, from the feel of water on your body, to the smells of soap and shampoo.[31]

Unplug—or not. Jonah Paquette, author of *Awestruck*, recommends unplugging from technology to become more present in our lives, which makes space for awe.[32] At the same time, though, technology opens up a world of awe to us. The internet is full of awe-inspiring videos of faraway lands we may never visit, microscopic miracles of nature, and breathtaking artistic performances.[33]

Spend time with a young child. Everything is novel and mysterious to children. They can help you see the world through their eyes and increase your own feelings of awe at the simple wonders that we adults often take for granted.

Read the biography of someone who inspires you. Remember, other people's goodness is the most common source of awe!

Visit an art, history, or science museum to encounter new and mind-bending displays. If you can't make it out, Amster and Eagle suggest treating your own home like a museum.[34] Observe the fine details of art, photographs, or sculptures in your space; look with fresh eyes at mirrors, lamps, rugs, and lights. Ponder what memories they bring up, and where all these items came from.

Sometimes, finding awe is more about how you pay attention than what you're paying attention to. So, keep an eye out for those experiences of chills, wide eyes, and wonder to find your awe moments.

For Diana Gameros, the Awe Outing helped her restore an emotional connection to Mexico after more than a decade of living in the United States and not seeing her homeland or her family.

Gameros wanted to carry that feeling of awe back to the United States with her, to incorporate it more in her daily life. So as an experiment, she decided to try the Awe Outing again, except this time while doing a mundane task she'd done countless times before—walking to her local grocery store.

Gameros slowed her pace, paying attention to her breath and surroundings, and the world seemed to slow down, too. Spring flowers looked brighter, leaves seemed thicker, an old woman smiled at her, and she smiled back with love. She felt connected on a deep level.

"It's amazing to realize that as soon as you turn off the phone and start breathing, how connected you become to the things that you see," says Gameros. "I was not exhausted and worried about my own thoughts, my chores. So I heard it all, and I saw it all. The Awe Outing was really important for me—to be fully present. I was happy. I was feeling alive."

Chapter 6

Mindfulness

Contributing coauthor: Haley Gray

Amy Schneider has an extraordinary ability to lock in and tune everything else out—it's why she was the first to hit the buzzer enough times on Jeopardy! to become the game show's highest-earning female champion, and the first openly trans contestant to make it to the Jeopardy! Tournament of Champions.

"There was such a good feeling about having that intense focus for periods of time," Schneider says.

But when her incredible run on the show was over, she discovered that sense of focus didn't translate to the other areas of her life—and when she signed a book deal, she really needed it to. "I've realized that I live so much in my mind and so little in my body," Schneider says. "It's been a real challenge to just sit down and put the rest of my thoughts out of my mind to write the book."

It wasn't just a lack of distraction she craved; she wanted calm, a sense of mental space so her creativity could flow. Schneider thought mindfulness might be the answer—but meditation had never worked for her before. So for our *Science of Happiness* podcast, she tried the Body Scan meditation, where you move your awareness from toe to head, letting go of passing thoughts by bringing your mind back to whatever sensations you notice in your body, cultivating acceptance for them.

The Body Scan made Schneider aware of the fact that, by focusing on sensations in her body, she was able to calm her mind.

"The mind and the body are not separable. They affect each other, and you can feel it actually happening," says Schneider. "When you relax your muscles, your mind gets less worried."

THE BENEFITS OF MINDFULNESS

Focusing on our breath. Slowing down enough to really taste our food. Noticing how fleeting our thoughts and feelings can be. These are all examples of being mindful, or bringing deliberate attention to our experience in the present moment through a gentle, nurturing lens—an important skill to develop for a happier life.

Mindfulness came out of a Buddhist meditation tradition and became more mainstream in the West when Jon Kabat-Zinn, a longtime Buddhist, offered his hospital patients secularized versions of mindfulness practices in an 8-week course he called Mindfulness-Based Stress Reduction (MBSR). Patients who learned and practiced skills like paying attention to their breath without judgment, focusing on bodily sensations, and mindful walking experienced reduced pain and suffering, ultimately leading to better health.[1]

This put mindfulness on Western scientists' radar and led to thousands of research studies supporting MBSR's benefits. More recently, researchers have also begun to look at the effects of individual practices and find ways that mindfulness practiced over a short period of time—whether that's a week or just a single session—can boost our well-being.

MINDFULNESS FOR STRESS

One of the most studied benefits of mindfulness is its effect on stress resilience. Several studies have found that people who train in mindfulness feel calmer and less stressed after facing challenges.[2] Even in high-stress situations, like working in an emergency room as a new intern or caregiving for someone with dementia, mindfulness helps people manage stress and reduce their chances of burning out.[3,4]

It may not take much to achieve these benefits. One recent study in Istanbul found that patients suffering chronic disease who tried out just three 20-minute sessions of mindful breathing reported lower symptoms of depression and stress compared to people relaxing quietly in a room.[5]

While a large part of mindfulness involves *noticing* our everyday experiences, the skill of *accepting* them without judgment may be even more influential on our well-being. In one study, researcher Emily Lindsay assigned one group to MBSR with an emphasis on accepting their experience in a nonjudgmental way, another group to MBSR without those instructions, and a last group to no mindfulness training. She and her team found that while all groups' stress dissipated over time, the group that went through MBSR with an acceptance emphasis experienced a much quicker, steeper decline in stress.

"Learning how to accept your present-moment experience is really important for reducing stress. It seems to be a key element of mindfulness training," says Lindsay.[6]

This was true for a study where university students did an ice water challenge. The students who were taught how to mindfully notice their breath and accept any feelings of pain or discomfort were able to keep their hand in cold water longer and felt less distress than those taught distraction techniques or told to do whatever they wanted to do.[7]

When we accept our thoughts and feelings rather than trying to push them away, it helps us cope better. If we become angry and mindfully recognize our feelings and thoughts without judgment, we can more easily understand what's going on inside of us and act accordingly. That may lead us to soothe ourselves and allow the anger to dissipate, rather than build up a head of steam and overreact by lashing out.[8,9]

MINDFULNESS FOR WELL-BEING AND PERFORMANCE

Mindfulness practices don't just calm our difficult emotions, though. They also seem to make us feel happier, healthier, and more resilient.[10,11] They can boost our immune systems, improve our sleep, help us age better, and reduce the pull of bad habits like alcohol use in recovering alcoholics and smartphone addiction.[12, 13, 14, 15, 16, 17]

When researchers looked at individual mindfulness practices,[18] they found that mindful breathing, body scans, loving-kindness meditation, and observing thoughts are all helpful for increasing people's positive feelings, energy, and focus on the present. We'll try some of these later in this chapter.

How do these benefits come about? Perhaps through improving our mental health. One study found that people suffering from anxiety and panic who trained in mindfulness meditation for 8 weeks felt less anxious in the short term, with improvements lasting at least three years.[19] There is even some evidence that mindfulness helps with depression and may prevent formerly depressed people from relapsing when it's combined with cognitive behavioral therapy.[20, 21]

Mindfulness can also help us focus and perform better in various environments.[22] One study found that women working in San Francisco and Seattle were less likely to have their attention hijacked if they went through a mindful breathing training; they stayed on task longer and felt better after work compared to employees who'd received relaxation training.[23] Likewise, schools offering mindfulness training have found that students pay better attention in class and seem more relaxed, and more mindful teachers are less likely to burn out.[24, 25]

This may be due to the way mindfulness reduces stress, but it may also be partly due to how mindfulness affects our brains.[26] Mindfulness has been found to change brain activity in ways that help people ignore distractions and pay better attention. Perhaps this is why more organizations are using mindfulness to improve people's performance and well-being—from classrooms to workplaces to prisons and even within the military.[27, 28, 29, 30]

MORE MINDFULNESS: HAPPIER RELATIONSHIPS

Being more mindful is good for our relationships too. One study found that couples randomly assigned to learn mindfulness skills over 8 weeks felt happier, less stressed in their relationships, and better able to cope with stress than those waiting for the training.[31] Mindfulness practices have been found to improve peer relationships among children and adolescents, too, which predicts their current and future well-being.[32]

Training in mindfulness may also help in conflict situations, making us more willing to apologize when we hurt others and resulting in more effective apologies.[33] Because mindfulness helps us see people as whole beings, with both good and bad qualities, it can decrease our negativity bias—the tendency to respond more to negative than positive information—when we interact with people from different races or groups, which can reduce stereotyping and prejudice.[34]

Though it's not totally clear why mindfulness has these social effects, it could be, as some research found, that more mindful people believe others can grow and change, which may help them be more flexible and optimistic about their relationships.[35] With attention, we can notice how everything in the world seems to shift and evolve over time, including the people around us, and be more accepting of how things are in the present. Or perhaps practicing mindfulness strengthens our sense of self and helps us act in ways more congruent with our values.[36, 37]

While mindfulness is certainly good for us as individuals, it's also important to note that mindfulness helps us act more altruistically in the face of suffering or unfairness—even when others may not.[38] One study found that Boston-based students trained in mindfulness who sat in a full waiting room were more likely to give up their seat to a person on crutches than students who hadn't done the training. Something about mindfulness helped them notice the need around them and want to take compassionate action.[39]

For all of these reasons, mindfulness is good for our happiness. Read on to find out how you can become more mindful yourself and reap its many rewards.

HOW MINDFUL ARE YOU?

Before we offer you mindfulness practices to try out, we'd like to give you the opportunity to reflect on your own experiences of mindfulness.[40] If you'd like, you can revisit these questions later to see if taking steps to practice mindfulness made a difference.

	Strongly disagree	Disagree	Neutral	Agree	Strongly agree
When I am startled, I notice what is going on inside my body.	1	2	3	4	5
I am aware of what thoughts are passing through my mind.	1	2	3	4	5
When someone asks how I am feeling, I can identify my emotions easily.	1	2	3	4	5
I tell myself that I shouldn't feel sad.	5	4	3	2	1
I wish I could control my emotions more easily.	5	4	3	2	1
I try to stay busy to keep thoughts or feelings from coming to mind.	5	4	3	2	1
When I walk outside, I am aware of smells or how the air feels against my face.	1	2	3	4	5
I notice changes inside my body, like my heart beating faster or my muscles getting tense.	1	2	3	4	5
Whenever my emotions change, I am conscious of them immediately.	1	2	3	4	5
When talking with other people, I am aware of their facial and body expressions.	1	2	3	4	5

Quick scoring guide: 10–30 = Low; 31–40 = Medium; 41–50 = High

MINDFULNESS PRACTICES

PRACTICE #1: BODY SCAN

Time: 5 minutes

The Body Scan is a type of meditation that involves focusing your attention on various parts of your body, and it can be performed while lying down, sitting, or in other postures. Research suggests that body scans can help calm an overactive mind and foster a sense of peace and happiness.[41, 42]

Especially for those new to the body scan, we recommend performing this practice with the audio from UCLA Mindful at ggia.berkeley.edu/practice/body_scan_meditation. However, you can also use the script below for guidance in doing the practice on your own.

Different people can respond differently to meditation practices, depending on considerations like past trauma or medical issues. Check in with yourself as you try out the two practices in this chapter, and listen to your body if you feel you need to shorten or end the practice.

- Begin by bringing your attention to your environment, slowly looking around and noticing that you are safe in this moment.
- Bring your attention into your body.
- You can close your eyes if that's comfortable for you, or maintain a soft gaze, with your eyes partially closed but not focusing on anything in particular.
- You can notice your body seated wherever you're seated, feeling the support of the chair or the floor beneath you.
- Take a few deep, long breaths, within the range of what is comfortable for you.
- As you take a deep breath, bring in more oxygen, enlivening the body. And as you exhale, you might experience a sense of relaxing more deeply.

- You can notice your feet on the floor, notice the sensations of your feet touching the floor: the weight, pressure, vibration, heat.
- You can notice your legs against the chair: pressure, pulsing, heaviness, lightness.
- Notice your back against the chair, supporting you. If you are not able to notice sensations in all areas of the body, that is okay. We are more connected to certain areas of the body than others at different times of the day.
- Bring your attention into your stomach area. If your stomach is tense or tight, can you allow it to soften? Take a breath.
- Notice your hands. Are your hands tense or tight? See if you can allow them to soften.
- Notice your arms. Feel any sensation in your arms. Do your best to allow your shoulders to be soft.
- Notice your neck and throat. Try to allow them to be soft. See if you can invite in a sense of relaxation.
- Try to soften your jaw. Do your best to allow your face and facial muscles to be soft.
- Now notice how your entire body is present. Take one more breath.
- Be aware of your whole body as well as you can. Take a breath.
- Slowly open up the eyes, without focusing on anything in particular. Allow the head and neck to gently rotate, taking in the space you are in. When you feel ready, you can return to your normal gaze.

How did it go? Was this the first time you tried a body scan meditation? Which parts of the meditation were difficult? Which were easier? What did you think and feel?

___

Pick a time and place to do another Body Scan this week.

My Body Scan plan:

___

PRACTICE #2: MINDFUL BREATHING

Time: 10 minutes

Mindful Breathing is a form of meditation in which you focus your attention on your breath—the inhalation and exhalation—and which can help with stress and emotion regulation.

You can do this practice while standing, but ideally you'll be sitting or even lying in a comfortable position. Your eyes may be open or closed, or you can maintain a soft gaze with your eyes partially closed but not focusing on anything in particular. It can help to set aside a designated time for this exercise, but it can also help to practice it when you're feeling particularly stressed or anxious. Experts believe regular practice can make mindful breathing easier to implement in difficult situations.

Sometimes, especially when trying to calm yourself in a stressful moment, it might help to start by taking an exaggerated breath: a deep inhale through your nostrils, hold your breath briefly, and a longer exhale through your mouth (one popular cadence is 4-7-8 seconds). Otherwise, observe each breath without trying to adjust it; it may help to focus on the rise and fall of your chest or the sensation through your nostrils. As you do so, you may find that your mind wanders, distracted by thoughts or bodily sensations; that's okay. You can notice that this is happening and try to gently bring your attention back to your breath.

Especially for those new to Mindful Breathing, we recommend performing this practice with the audio from UCLA Mindful[43] at ggia.berkeley.edu/practice/mindful_breathing. However, you can also use the script below for guidance in doing the practice on your own.

- Find a relaxed, comfortable position. You could be seated on a chair or on the floor on a cushion. Try to keep your back upright, but not too tight; hands resting wherever they're comfortable; tongue on the roof of your mouth or wherever it's comfortable.
- Notice and invite your body to relax. Allow yourself to become curious about your body—the sensations it experiences, the touch, the connection with the floor or the chair. Do your best to relax any areas of tightness or tension. Breathe.
- Tune into the rhythm of your breath. You can feel the natural flow of breath—in, out. You don't need to do anything to your breath. Not long, not short, but natural. Notice where you feel your breath in your body. It might be in your abdomen. It may be in your chest or

throat or in your nostrils. See if you can feel the sensations of breath, one breath at a time. When one breath ends, the next breath begins. If you are not able to notice the breath in all areas of the body, that's okay. We are more connected to certain areas of the body than others at different times of the day.

- As you do this, you might notice that your mind starts to wander; you may start thinking about other things. If this happens, it's not a problem; it's very natural. Try to notice that your mind has wandered. You can say "thinking" or "wandering" in your head softly. And then gently redirect your attention back to the breathing.
- Stay here for 5 to 7 minutes. Notice your breath in silence. From time to time, you'll get lost in thought; then return to your breath.
- After a few minutes, once again notice your body, your whole body, seated here. Let yourself relax even more deeply and then, if it's possible for you, please offer yourself some appreciation for doing this practice today.

What did Mindful Breathing feel like for you? Were you able to catch your mind wandering away from your breath?

_____
_____
_____
_____
_____

Pick a time and place to do Mindful Breathing again this week.

My Mindful Breathing plan:

_____

_____

_____

_____

PUTTING MINDFULNESS INTO PRACTICE

We've shared just two mindfulness practices, but there are countless others you can find online or at your local meditation center.

In the realm of formal meditation, which practice is best for you? Research has found that different practices have different benefits, depending on whether you're focusing on your breathing, paying attention to your body, cultivating warm and positive feelings, or observing your own thoughts.[44] Simple breathing meditation might be more helpful for regulating your emotions and becoming less judgmental, while loving-kindness meditation could be useful for working with guilt or fostering kinder thoughts toward others.[45][46] In fact, studies find that different types of meditation lead to changes in different areas of the brain.[47]

Researcher Hooria Jazaieri, who has run compassion and mindfulness trainings, offers some tips for finding what works for you:

> *My recommendations . . . are to try out different durations, types, and frequencies of meditation and jot down how you feel before and after the practice. It's even important to experiment with different times of the day (I recommend that you do the practice before you "need it"). Making time to intentionally reflect on your experiences with the practices is key. For*

> *some people, meditating for 20–30 minutes a day is not fitting—the only way to find out what's right for you is to experiment.*

It could be helpful to intersperse short meditation practices throughout your day, rather than feeling you need to carve out an hour in the morning or evening. Workplace experts Rasmus Hougaard and Jacqueline Carter recommend habits like taking a 10-minute pause in your car or at your desk before your workday begins, meditating briefly before or at the start of meetings, and using your commute home as a moment to just *be*.[48]

When you start to practice, you might struggle with creating new habits and staying motivated. As researcher Carly Hunt writes, "New meditators often question whether meditation will in fact be beneficial, doubt whether they're meditating correctly, struggle to find space and time for practice, and sense that meditation conflicts with their cultural or familial norms."[49] That last piece refers to people worrying that their family might find meditation odd or that it doesn't fit in with their religion.

She suggests finding a meditation group as a way to stay accountable and get support. It can also be helpful to keep in mind both the science-based benefits of mindfulness, like the ones we cover in this chapter, and your personal reason for practicing—whether that's "to live life more fully, be less emotionally reactive, or offer more compassion to others," Hunt writes. Once you start to see benefits for yourself, such as a sense of calm or meaning, she suggests paying special attention to them—they may be the fuel to help you keep practicing.

INFORMAL MINDFULNESS

Kabat-Zinn emphasizes that although mindfulness can be cultivated through formal meditations, that's not the only way. "It's not really about sitting in the full lotus, like pretending you're a statue in a British museum," he says. "It's about living your life as if it really mattered, moment by moment by moment by moment."[50]

Like some other teachers, researcher and mindfulness trainer Leah

Weiss calls this *mindfulness in action*: "becoming mindfully aware of your thoughts, feelings, and surroundings even while you're engaged in some other activity."[51]

Here are a few key tips that Kabat-Zinn, Jazaieri, Weiss, and others offer to help you incorporate mindfulness into your days:

- Pay close attention to your breathing, especially when you're feeling intense emotions. For example, spend a few minutes breathing quietly when you wake up, before you get out of bed.
- Notice—really notice—what you're sensing in a given moment: the sights, sounds, and smells that ordinarily slip by without reaching your conscious awareness. One fun study found that mindful dishwashing—being conscious of the breath, aware of the fact that you are washing dishes—can make us feel more inspired and less nervous[52]; you could try being mindful as you brush your teeth or eat your lunch.
- Tune into your body's physical sensations, from the water hitting your skin in the shower to the way your body rests in a chair.
- Tune in to your own intentions in a given moment. For example, in a meeting, maybe you're hoping to improve your relationship with one of your colleagues. On a walk or at dinner, maybe you're intending to truly rest and connect with those around you.
- Communicate with mindfulness: Be aware of any fears you have around pleasing others or protecting your reputation, and aim to share in an authentic way.
- Notice when your mind wanders to the past or future, and bring it back to something in the present—your breath, your body, or your environment.
- Shift from judging to observing: Notice if you have a tendency to label yourself and others as good or bad, lazy or boring. See what it would feel like to let go of judgments and just observe people and situations.

- Set a mindful password for one of your accounts—a word or phrase that reminds you to be present—or hang a picture or sign that reminds you of mindfulness.

Students from our Science of Happiness course really noticed how applying awareness to the details of everyday life enhanced their joy and appreciation. Christophe Watelet from Belgium says, "For me, meditation is about gradually slowing down the pace in one's life and beginning to enjoy the simple things." For Yanna Papaioannou from the U.K., mindfulness is about listening, pausing, and savoring. "I try and practice daily, whether I'm enjoying a cup of coffee, admiring my blossoming orchid, the smell of a sandalwood-scented candle burning, watching a robin pick a worm from the bird feeder outside my patio, or enjoying a conversation with a group of close friends sitting in a café."

Mindfulness is one of the most popular skills we share in this workbook, having exploded into mainstream media, workplace programs, apps, and more. With that in mind, all of us could be forgiven for thinking mindfulness is the solution to all our problems—but, of course, it's not.

At times, and for certain people, practicing mindfulness may actually make us less happy. Because it asks us to look deep within ourselves, it's best approached gently and perhaps with the guidance of a skillful teacher.

"At times, sitting quietly with oneself can be a difficult—even painful—experience," explains Jazaieri. "For individuals who have experienced some sort of trauma, sitting and meditating can at times bring up recent or sometimes decades-old painful memories and experiences that they may not be prepared to confront."

At its best, though, mindfulness can help us truly tune into our positive experiences, enhancing the joy of gratitude or the warmth of kindness. And when we suffer, it helps us sit with our suffering without insisting it be different. With a little mindfulness, we become present to our experiences, to ourselves, and to those around us, so we don't miss out on the moments of our lives.

A year after trying the Body Scan meditation for our podcast, Amy

Schneider published her book *In the Form of a Question: The Rewards and Joys of a Curious Life.* Having a set of steps to follow in order to feel both present and embodied is what made mindfulness work for her, and aided her book-writing process.

"This was a way of getting some of those benefits while still having a script to go through in my mind to keep me focused," says Schneider. "Once I came out of that Body Scan, all the different thoughts that have been running around in my head, they all quieted down."

Chapter 7
Gratitude

It was during Kai Koerber's senior year of high school, on Valentine's Day 2018. He was in the middle of guitar class when a shooter opened fire. He texted his mother, "Something is happening at my school. I'm not sure, but I just want to let you know that if anything happens to me, that I love you."

Koerber survived, but 17 students and staff members at Marjory Stoneman Douglas High School in Parkland, Florida, were killed that day. Koerber, and countless others, were traumatized. Fortunately for Koerber, he had a strong foundation to support him—his mother.

She motivated him to use the unwanted spotlight on his high school to protest gun violence. She helped him start a nonprofit, Societal Reform Corporation, to raise money and advocate for mental health and mindfulness education in schools. She encouraged him to study hard, and he went on to get a degree in computer science from UC Berkeley.

"She really put forward this energy that things are gonna be all right," says Koerber. "And I'm going to be the captain of my own soul. That's really something that she would express to me every day, in more ways than one."

Koerber was deeply thankful for his mother, and he wanted to express that in a meaningful and impactful way. So Koerber wrote her a Gratitude Letter, which he shared with her and also on our *Science of Happiness* podcast. It was a small gesture to show his boundless gratitude.

"My mother was really there for me professionally and personally," says Koerber. "She's my best friend, because there is nobody else I could talk to about the things that I experienced and the things I want to see going forward in my life besides my mother. I couldn't ask for anyone better."

THE BENEFITS OF GRATITUDE

Even when very bad things happen to us, it can help to stop for a moment and pay attention to the good in our lives too. Whether it's having clean air to breathe, an educated mind, a healthy body, a neighborhood park, friends, or mothers who love us, we can see these good things as gifts or blessings that have come to us, in part, from something or someone outside of ourselves. If we don't notice these good things—if we take them for granted or don't even register them—we can be left with a skewed view of the world.

That's where practicing gratitude can help. Without ignoring the bad, we can turn our attention to the gifts in our lives and give thanks to those responsible for providing them. Cultivating gratitude can lead to greater happiness, filling us with warm feelings and a sense of connection to others.[1] Even in the most difficult circumstances, like what Koerber suffered at Parkland that day, taking some time to focus on what we're grateful for can help us get through it.

GOOD FOR MENTAL AND PHYSICAL HEALTH

There are many studies showing how having a grateful outlook on life can lead to greater well-being.[2] In one seminal study by gratitude researcher Robert Emmons, young adults who wrote about things they were grateful for once a week for 10 weeks—the Gratitude Journal exercise you'll find later in the chapter—experienced better moods, felt more optimistic, and slept better than those who wrote about their daily lives.[3] People who feel more grateful also tend to have a stronger sense of social connection and meaning in life.[4]

Though gratitude can make us feel better in everyday life, it's also helpful when things are going poorly. People who are more grateful tend to cope better with grief, feel more supported when facing breast cancer, and have greater quality of life when living with multiple sclerosis.[5, 6, 7] Gratitude has even helped people recover from trauma incurred from natural disasters and from living under violent political conflict.[8]

One study found that young adults who tended to be more grateful prior to the COVID-19 pandemic suffered less anxiety, had stronger social connections, and maintained a more positive outlook on life after the pandemic started—all of which helped protect their mental health during that trying time.[9] Gratitude seems to help us cope better by guiding us to reframe negative experiences in more positive ways, which makes us more resilient.[10]

As Emmons writes, "In the face of demoralization, gratitude has the power to energize. In the face of brokenness, gratitude has the power to heal. In the face of despair, gratitude has the power to bring hope."[11]

Research suggests that feeling grateful at work may have benefits, too.[14] These might include less stress and fewer health complaints, as well as a greater sense that we can achieve our goals. Though it's not clear why gratitude helps in these ways, one study found that people in South Korea nudged to feel grateful as opposed to resentful exhibited brain activation suggesting they felt less anxiety, ruminated less, and were better able to manage difficult emotions.[15]

GRATITUDE IN OUR RELATIONSHIPS

Gratitude is a quintessential social emotion, as it makes us feel closer and more connected to others. Romantic partners who feel grateful and exchange words of appreciation are more likely to stay together.[16] Also, when one partner suffers from an insecure attachment—where they fear being abandoned and are more needy and clingy—receiving gratitude can help soothe them and make them feel happier in the relationship.

With a friend, expressing gratitude simultaneously benefits the recipient and can also make us more invested in the friendship.[17] Expressing gratitude can help our relationships with our children, too, even if our gratitude isn't directed toward them. Parents in the United States who were randomly assigned to write a gratitude letter to someone they felt grateful for experienced greater well-being and felt closer to their children (and more satisfaction with parenting) 1 week later in comparison to parents who journaled about their general activities.[18]

While the ability to express gratitude may not emerge immediately in life, children as young as 4 years old prefer others who seem grateful—and they are more likely to share resources with a grateful person than an ungrateful one.[19] Grateful adolescents tend to feel better and more connected to their schools and teachers—even those from less resourced, high-risk communities.[20, 21] And, in one study in Spain, adolescents assigned to learn about and practice gratitude through journaling were less likely to engage in cyberbullying.[22] These and other studies suggest that gratitude may have evolved as a means of strengthening social networks and forming more caring, cooperative communities.

Indeed, grateful people tend to be kinder and more altruistic than others—including toward strangers, not just people they know.[23] In another study, people who were guided to feel grateful spent more time in a tedious task to help out someone else—filling out a long and boring survey—when given the opportunity.[24]

Research by Sonja Lyubomirsky and Christina Armenta suggests this may be due to how gratitude helps us be better people, in general—humbler, more interested in self-improvement, and more inspired to act morally.[25] Interestingly, expressing or receiving gratitude can have a ripple effect, so that people who witness us being grateful or receiving gratitude will want to help out others themselves.[26]

All of this suggests that gratitude not only makes us happier, but also has the important function of helping us create a more compassionate world. If you'd like to try practicing more gratitude in your own life, read on.

HOW GRATEFUL ARE YOU?

Before we offer you gratitude practices to try out, we'd like to give you the opportunity to reflect on your own experiences of gratitude.[27] If you'd like, you can revisit these questions later to see if taking steps to practice gratitude made a difference.

	Strongly disagree	Disagree	Neutral	Agree	Strongly agree
I feel very thankful for my degree of physical health.	1	2	3	4	5
I count my blessings for what I have in this world.	1	2	3	4	5
I reflect on the worst times in my life to help me realize how fortunate I am now.	1	2	3	4	5
It is important to appreciate things such as health, family, and friends.	1	2	3	4	5
I really notice and acknowledge the good things I get in life.	1	2	3	4	5
I am content with what I have.	1	2	3	4	5
I remind myself how fortunate I am to have the privileges and opportunities I have encountered in life.	1	2	3	4	5
I remind myself to think about the good things I have in my life.	1	2	3	4	5

	Strongly disagree	Disagree	Neutral	Agree	Strongly agree
I appreciate my degree of success in life so far.	1	2	3	4	5
When I see someone less fortunate than myself, I realize how lucky I am.	1	2	3	4	5

Quick scoring guide: 10–30 = Low; 31–40 = Medium; 41–50 = High

GRATITUDE PRACTICES

PRACTICE #1: GRATITUDE JOURNAL

Time: 15 minutes

Gratitude journaling has been tested around the world, from Brazil to Turkey to Malaysia. Research suggests that this simple practice of recording instances of goodness in your life can be beneficial for your well-being, emotional life, and physical health.

There's no wrong way to keep a gratitude journal, but here are some guidelines to help you get started.

In the space below, write down up to five things for which you feel grateful. The physical record is important—don't just do this exercise in your head. The things you list can be relatively small in importance ("The tasty sandwich I had for lunch today") or relatively large ("My sister gave birth to a healthy baby boy"). The goal of the exercise is to remember a good event, experience, person, or thing in your life—then enjoy the good emotions that come with it.

As you write, here are some important tips:

1. **Be as specific as possible.** Being as clear as possible is key to fostering gratitude. "I'm grateful that my coworkers brought me soup when I was sick on Tuesday" may be more effective than "I'm grateful for my coworkers."

2. **Go for depth over breadth.** Going into detail about a particular person or thing for which you're grateful carries more benefits than a surface-level list of many things.
3. **Get personal.** Focusing on people to whom you are grateful has more of an impact than focusing on things.
4. **Remember what might have been.** Be grateful for the negative outcomes you avoided, escaped, prevented, or turned into something positive—try not to take that good fortune for granted.
5. **See good things as gifts.** Thinking of the good things in your life as gifts helps you avoid taking them for granted. Try to enjoy and savor the gifts you've received.
6. **Savor surprises.** Try to record events that were unexpected or surprising, as these tend to bring up stronger feelings of gratitude.
7. **Aim for variety.** Writing about some of the same people and things is okay, but try to focus on different details each time you write about them.
8. **Write regularly.** Whether you write daily or weekly, commit to a regular time to journal. Do your best to honor that commitment.

I'm grateful for:
_____
_____
_____
_____
_____
_____
_____

When will you try Gratitude Journaling again? Where will you write—in a notebook, in your phone's notes application, or on your computer?

My Gratitude Journal plan:

_____

_____

_____

_____

PRACTICE #2: GRATITUDE LETTER

Time: 10 minutes

The Gratitude Letter, a longer message of gratitude to a particular person, has been found to be one of the most beneficial gratitude practices, helping people feel happier for up to a month or two later.[28, 29]

When Koerber began to write a Gratitude Letter to his mom, he thought about how she had been a young, single mother who persevered in order to give her son a good life, and how she'd shown him how to find light after darkness. But it was hard to translate that gratitude into words at first.

"Being a student, you're used to writing things that are scholarly and with the utmost etiquette," says Koerber. "But [the Gratitude Letter] helped me break down those walls."

Koerber's letter to his mother read, in part:

"Dear Ma, thank you is how every letter I write to you should begin. Thank you for loving me before I knew what love was. You taught me what it is to believe and hold love in your heart, even when the world shows you evil. Thank you for picking me up when the world kicked me down."

Koerber shared the letter with his mother, and it filled her with a deep gratitude and sense of connection to her son. And, in line with research suggesting gratitude has a snowball effect, she later responded with a Gratitude Letter of her own, sharing her love for her son.

"[The Gratitude Letter] was a chance to reconnect with myself so I could put pen to paper and really express how grateful I am for all the things that my mother has done for me," says Koerber. "Even before I was cognizant enough to know she was doing them. It was definitely an experience I'll never forget."

To start your own Gratitude Letter, call to mind someone who did something for you for which you are extremely grateful but to whom you may have never expressed your deep gratitude. This could be a relative, friend, teacher, or colleague. Try to pick someone who is still alive and could meet you face-to-face in the next week. It may be most helpful to select a person or act that you haven't thought about for a while—something that isn't always on your mind.

Now, write a letter to one of these people, guided by the following steps.

- Write directly to this person, as if you are speaking to them.
- Don't worry about grammar or spelling.
- Describe in specific terms what they did, why you are grateful to them, and how their behavior affected your life. Try to be as concrete as possible.
- Describe what you are doing in your life now and how you often remember their efforts.

Dear _____,
_____
_____
_____
_____
_____
_____

Next, try if at all possible to deliver your letter in person, following these steps:

- Plan a visit with the recipient. Let that person know you'd like to see them and have something special to share, but don't reveal the exact purpose of the meeting.
- When you meet, let the person know that you are grateful to them and would like to read a letter expressing your gratitude; ask that they refrain from interrupting until you're done.
- Take your time reading the letter. While you read, pay attention to their reaction as well as your own.
- After you have read the letter, be receptive to their reaction and discuss your feelings together.
- Remember to give the letter to the person when you leave.

If physical distance keeps you from making a visit, you may choose to arrange a phone or video chat.

> **KEEP IN MIND**
>
> Cross-cultural research suggests that writing Gratitude Letters may be less beneficial for people from certain collectivist cultures.
>
> Some studies suggest that South Koreans and Asian Americans who write Gratitude Letters don't see as many benefits for their well-being as Anglo Americans.[30, 31]
>
> Other studies have found that Indian and Taiwanese people don't feel more grateful after writing Gratitude Letters.[32]
>
> Expressing appreciation for other people's help may generate more mixed emotions for these groups, like indebtedness, guilt, sadness, and regret.[33, 34, 35] One Indian participant in a study wrote, "[The] only thing which always pulls me down is that I could have given some gift as a token of gratitude."
>
> One way to stave off feelings of indebtedness, says researcher Liudmila Titova, is to imagine, if you're able, that whatever help or kindness you received was given freely.

PUTTING GRATITUDE INTO PRACTICE

Gratitude is ultimately about recognizing the good things in our lives, and not letting them slip by unnoticed. Sometimes we might do that naturally, but other times our brains need a little help. If you'd like to nudge your mind in a more grateful direction, here are a few things you can try.

Imagine an alternate universe. Pick someone or something you'd like to summon up some gratitude for—maybe a spouse or friend, a job or trip. Then, think about all the tiny decisions, random events, and luck that had to happen for you to meet them or have that particular experience. Maybe you wouldn't have met your spouse if you hadn't taken up pickleball rather than tennis, moved out of the city, or decided to stop at the grocery store one night. Imagine a life without this person or experience and all the benefits and joys you wouldn't have. Then, remember how things actually turned out and what it has meant to you.

Abstain. One of the biggest obstacles to gratitude is habituation, how we get used to positive experiences so they no longer pack the same punch. To get unhabituated, pick something you enjoy regularly and freely—like a food or drink, or TV watching—and give it up for a week. Once you're able to indulge again, you might feel a burst of spontaneous gratitude.

Savor. Savoring, the practice of being aware of good feelings to help enhance them, is halfway between a gratitude and a mindfulness practice. One great gateway to savoring is by using our senses of touch, sight, smell, taste, and hearing—to smell cookies baking or feel the warmth of sunlight on our faces. Little rituals can help slow us down and shift our attention toward the good in the present moment,[36] like gazing out the window every morning as you drink your coffee or clinking a "cheers" before a meal.

Take in the good. Psychologist Rick Hanson, who likes to say that our brains act like Velcro for the bad and Teflon for the good, suggests staying with positive experiences for a little longer than you would normally—from 5 to 20 seconds. "Actively look for good news, particularly the little stuff of daily life: the faces of children, the smell of an orange, a memory from a happy vacation, a minor success at work," he writes.[37] As you marinate in the goodness, imagine absorbing it into your mind, body, and heart.

Express your thanks. Many gratitude practices can be done in solitude, so it's easy to forget one of the simplest ways to practice gratitude: Say thank you! On our gratitude journaling website Thnx4.org, people felt that their gratitude experience had a stronger impact on their day—closer to making their whole day glorious than just making them smile momentarily—if they actually expressed their thanks.[38]

Keep the focus on others. Along with forgetting to express our gratitude, sometimes we can take gratitude too far as a *self*-improvement exercise and forget what it's really about, says Emmons: other people. If you're obsessing about how grateful you are and whether you're feeling grateful enough, he says you're practicing "to-do list gratitude"—yet another item on your long slog of daily tasks.[39]

Instead, we should think about gratitude as a way of looking at the world and recognizing all the good things that come to us from outside ourselves. One way to do that is to keep an eye out for people's kindness and good intentions. Pay special attention when someone uses their time and energy to make your life better—whether it's a stranger letting you cut in front of them in the checkout line or a friend sending you a book recommendation just because.

Go through the motions. Experts believe that it's the repeated practice of gratitude—even when we don't *feel* grateful—that will eventually lead to a more enduring attitude of gratitude. "If you go through grateful motions, the emotion of gratitude should be triggered," writes Emmons.[40]

GRATITUDE IN HARD TIMES

Sometimes, when we struggle with gratitude, it's because the difficulties in life are weighing us down—so much so that we wonder how it's even possible to feel grateful at all.

In those moments, the first thing to know is that there's no obligation to feel anything other than what we're feeling.

One of our Science of Happiness students, Amanda Clarke from Australia, knows this firsthand. Years ago, she suffered a stroke without knowing it, which took months to diagnose. "When I was told what had happened, I went through a number of different emotions—grief, anger, sadness," she recalls. "Quite a few people told me I should be so grateful that I was alive, and not disabled, but I just couldn't get there for a long time." For her, it took about 2 years to get to a sense of gratitude:

> *Gradually, incrementally almost, I found gratitude by noticing a few small things each day, like the feeling of swimming at the beach, or a kookaburra singing in the front yard, and I could be grateful for these small things. Now, almost 4 years later, I feel very grateful for my life and my health. I have never quite understood why this took so long, but I don't feel angry at myself. I just felt the emotions that were present during my recovery and accepted that the movement to gratitude was a slow one.*

If you're drawn to gratitude as a way to cope in hard times, Emmons suggests taking a gentle attitude.[41] In other words, don't force yourself to feel grateful, but just try practicing a little and see what happens. He recommends asking yourself:

- What lessons did the experience teach me?
- What ability did the experience draw out of me that surprised me?
- How am I now more the person I want to be because of it?
- Have my challenging feelings about the experience limited or prevented my ability to feel gratitude in the time since it occurred?
- Has the experience removed a personal obstacle that previously prevented me from feeling grateful?[42]

It's very possible that the difficulties we're going through today will inspire gratitude in the future—something we can look back on to help us remember how far we've come.

EMBRACING OUR INTERDEPENDENCE

Gratitude alerts us to goodness, but it also highlights something else that might make us a little uneasy: our reliance on each other.

"Gratitude requires you to be vulnerable," says researcher Todd Kashdan[43]:

> *You essentially have to acknowledge the fact that you cannot get through life without the benefits and the gifts and the strengths and the social resources and the intellectual resources of other people.... You have to admit that you are not whole without other people.*

For some, that might be comforting; for others, a little unsettling. The solution, says Kashdan, is to let people be kind to you, to allow them the fulfillment of doing something nice for someone else. And just say thank you.

Chapter 8

Self-Compassion

Contributing coauthor: Haley Gray

René Brooks was a smart kid. At school, she was identified as *gifted*, and that label came with high expectations. But she seemed to always be getting into trouble, and constantly disappointing the people around her.

As an adult, those feelings intensified. What Brooks didn't know was that she had undiagnosed attention deficit disorder, or ADHD.

Things like misplacing an invitation to an important family event—a common occurrence for someone with ADHD—could leave her loved ones feeling she didn't really care and Brooks feeling terrible.

"I would think, 'You're just selfish. You think you can do whatever you want. You don't care. You're messy. You're lazy.' It's easy to internalize those types of messages," she says.

Brooks says being diagnosed at 25 was liberating.[1] She finally understood why these things kept happening to her. But all those years of criticism had left an indelible mark; she couldn't seem to escape her relentless inner critic. So for our *Science of Happiness* podcast, Brooks tried an exercise in writing herself a Self-Compassionate Letter, with warm and kind messages, using the same tone she would for a dear friend.

At first, writing didn't come naturally to her.

"I am super cynical when it comes to practices like this," says Brooks. "When you're trying to run from systemic racism and you're trying to survive micro-aggressions in every place of your life, there's not a lot of time for this kind of self-compassion."

But she pushed herself to try it anyway and realized that what had at first seemed rote and corny was actually extremely useful to her. The Self-Compassionate Letter gave Brooks a structure to practice self-kindness: It was a concrete thing she could easily carve out a few minutes for.

"It sounds cheesy to write a letter for yourself," Brooks says. "It wasn't."

THE BENEFITS OF SELF-COMPASSION

There are all kinds of suffering we might experience in life. Sometimes, we feel stressed, rejected, lonely, or wronged. Other times, we make mistakes—like missing an important appointment, failing at our jobs, or letting a loved one down—and we feel shame or guilt for our perceived failures.

How do you treat yourself in those moments? If we have a harsh inner critic, we may beat ourselves up about what we did, or believe there's something wrong with us for the way we feel. But this can hurt our well-being and keep us stuck in life. This is where self-compassion can offer a better way forward.

Like its cousin compassion, self-compassion involves us recognizing suffering and offering kindness, but, in this case, we're the recipient. Self-compassion is treating ourselves as a best friend would, with understanding, warmth, and clear-eyed wisdom.

Researcher Kristin Neff, who pioneered self-compassion research in Western psychology, says it involves three main components: mindful awareness of our thoughts and feelings, self-directed messages of kindness, and a sense of shared humanity—meaning, a recognition that all beings suffer and no one is perfect. By practicing self-compassion, we tame rather than avoid our inner critic, offer ourselves kindness when we're hurting, and stay more open to learning and growth.

HOW SELF-COMPASSION CAN IMPROVE YOUR LIFE

Self-compassion is related to but different from self-esteem, which is more about maintaining a positive self-image. While both have their benefits, practicing self-compassion can help us have a more stable sense of self-worth in the face of challenges.[2] And, as one study found, people who are more self-compassionate endure stressful circumstances better and have less anxiety than those with high levels of self-esteem.[3]

In another study, undergraduate women students were randomly assigned to either practice self-compassion or learn more about the power of attention (or neither) before a stressful task—making an oral presentation before a pair of unfriendly evaluators. In comparison to the other groups, the self-compassion group recovered better from the test-induced stress and felt less anxiety, both in their own minds and according to measurements of their physiology.[4]

Similarly, other studies have found that people who are more self-compassionate recover better after enduring situations that might hurt their sense of self—such as facing discrimination due to their sexual or gender identification or dealing with PTSD after returning from active-duty combat.[5,6]

Self-compassion is tied to better mental health in other situations, too, with potential benefits for people at risk for substance abuse, with body image issues, or suffering depression.[7,8,9] In one experiment, people in Germany diagnosed with major depression were induced to feel depressed four different times, then assigned to either wait, accept their uncomfortable feelings, take a different perspective on their situation, or practice self-compassion to try to feel better. Overall, those who used self-compassion improved their mood as much as those in the acceptance and perspective groups (two common tools for treating depressive moods). And self-compassion was the most beneficial strategy for the most depressed patients.[10]

Self-compassion may promote resilience during difficult times because more self-compassionate people tend to use healthier coping strategies (e.g., seeking emotional support) and avoid unhealthier strategies (e.g., excessive ruminating or self-blame). Perhaps that's why researchers found that more self-compassionate people in Greece experienced better mental health and greater happiness during the COVID-19 pandemic.[11]

In addition, being more self-compassionate is generally good for relationships.[12] It helps us be less defensive so we can see another person's point of view and compromise without subordinating our own needs, thus creating more relationship harmony.[13] Romantic couples who are more self-compassionate are less likely to repress or ruminate over difficult feelings and can offer more caring, supportive communication to each other.[14]

Self-compassionate people may also be more tolerant of those who are different from them. As one study found, among university students who were mostly female and mostly Hispanic or white, those who were more self-compassionate felt more warmly toward homeless people, senior citizens, and Asians. They also rated people from those groups as more competent than less self-compassionate students did. This seemed to be due to the stronger sense of common humanity that self-compassion encourages.[15]

WHY PEOPLE MAY RESIST SELF-COMPASSION

Despite these benefits, you may be wary of offering yourself compassion. You might find self-compassion distasteful or indicative of weakness, equating it with self-pity, self-indulgence, or just plain self-centeredness.

But, according to Neff, self-compassion is none of those things. Instead, it is a powerful way to tap into what we already know but too often forget: that life can be hard, and we all make mistakes we regret and struggle at times. It's part of being human.

"The feeling that certain things 'shouldn't' be happening makes us feel both shamed and isolated," she writes. "At those times, remembering that we aren't really alone in our suffering—that hardship and struggle are deeply embedded in the human condition—can make a radical difference."[16]

Some people object to self-compassion because they think it means letting themselves or someone else off the hook, rather than taking responsibility for mistakes or poor judgment. But research suggests the contrary: Self-compassionate people are *more* likely to admit to wrongdoing and try to make amends than less self-compassionate people.[17] Self-compassion actually protects our self-efficacy (i.e., a sense of control over our own lives) in the face of failure, which can help us persevere.[18]

Why? When we don't habitually criticize ourselves or beat ourselves up, it makes sense that we are more willing to take a look at things we might not like about ourselves. Instead of the sting of shame or self-judgment, we experience warm feelings of support that help motivate us to change and improve.[19]

For all of these reasons, it seems that self-compassion is good for our overall well-being—in both everyday life and in difficult circumstances.[20] Fortunately, self-compassion can also be cultivated. Read on to find out how.

HOW SELF-COMPASSIONATE ARE YOU?

Before we offer you self-compassion practices to try out, we'd like to give you the opportunity to reflect on your own experiences of self-compassion.[21] If you'd like, you can revisit these questions later to see if taking steps to practice self-compassion made a difference.

	Strongly disagree	Disagree	Neutral	Agree	Strongly agree
I try to be patient and understanding toward the aspects of my personality that I don't like.	1	2	3	4	5
When I'm feeling down, I tend to obsess and fixate on everything that's wrong.	5	4	3	2	1
When things are going badly for me, I see the difficulties as part of life that everyone goes through.	1	2	3	4	5

When I fail at something important to me, I become consumed by feelings of inadequacy.	5	4	3	2	1
When I'm feeling down, I try to approach my feelings with curiosity and openness.	1	2	3	4	5
When I'm down and out, I remind myself that there are lots of other people in the world feeling as I do.	1	2	3	4	5
When times are really difficult, I tend to be tough on myself.	5	4	3	2	1
When something upsets me, I try to keep my emotions in balance.	1	2	3	4	5
I try to see my failings as part of the human condition.	1	2	3	4	5
I'm kind to myself when I'm experiencing suffering.	1	2	3	4	5

Quick scoring guide: 10–30 = Low; 31–40 = Medium; 41–50 = High

SELF-COMPASSION PRACTICES

PRACTICE #1: SELF-COMPASSIONATE LETTER

Time: 15 minutes

Like an encouraging note from a friend, the Self-Compassionate Letter from researcher Kristin Neff helps you give yourself the warmth and encouragement that you need. Research finds that people who write Self-Compassionate Letters daily for a week feel happier and less depressed up to 3 months later.[22]

To try the practice, think of something about yourself that makes you feel mildly ashamed, insecure, or not good enough. It could be something related to your personality, behavior, abilities, relationships, or any other part of your life.

Once you choose something, reflect on how it makes you feel. Sad? Embarrassed? Angry? The next step is to write a letter from yourself, to yourself, expressing compassion, understanding, and acceptance for this part of yourself with which you struggle.

As you express your thoughts and feelings in the letter, try to be kind to yourself and be as honest as possible. Write whatever comes to you, but try to write in a way that makes you feel nurtured and soothed. Keep in mind that no one but you will see your letter, and there is no right or wrong way of doing this exercise. You can spend anywhere from 5 to 15 minutes writing.

> "It felt good to cut myself some slack and to recognize that my experience was a human experience. I felt more connected to the world, in general, and felt more optimistic that I could improve, as opposed to feeling down on myself, and like there is no hope for me." —Science of Happiness student Aparna Sankararaman

As you write the letter, follow these guidelines:
1. Imagine that there is someone who loves and accepts you unconditionally for who you are. What would that person say to you about this part of yourself? Think about what you would say to a friend in your position or what a friend would say to you in this situation.
2. Remind yourself that everyone has things about themselves that they don't like and that nobody is perfect. Think about how many other people in the world might be struggling with the same thing with which you're struggling.

3. Consider the ways in which events that have happened in your life, the family environment you grew up in, or even your genetic makeup may have contributed to this thing about yourself that you dislike.
4. In a compassionate way, ask yourself whether there are things you could do to improve or better cope with this part of you. Focus on how positive changes could make you feel happier, healthier, or more fulfilled. Try to avoid judging yourself.
5. After writing the letter, put it out of sight for a little while. Then come back to it later and read it again. It may be especially helpful to read it whenever you're feeling bad about this part of yourself, as a reminder to be more self-compassionate.

Dear _____ ,

_____

_____

_____

_____

René Brooks knows very well that shame and blame are not good motivators. She started to coach others with a business she dubbed "Black Girl, Lost Keys," helping other women let go of the shame around ADHD so they can live healthier, more fulfilling lives.

"It's a process to unlearn immediately jumping to shame when you're unhappy with something you've done," Brooks says.

The Self-Compassionate Letter gave her a way to move forward: Instead of facing down the larger-than-life task of completely eliminating negative self-talk, this writing practice was something Brooks could slip into her schedule to remind her to be kind to herself. It also gave her a practical way to change her tone—by speaking to herself the way she would to someone she was coaching.

"Some of us only know how to motivate ourselves through negativity, like shame and blame and anger," Brooks says. "[The Self-Compassionate Letter] can be a starting point for seeing what you need to replace those things with instead."

PRACTICE #2: HOW WOULD YOU TREAT A FRIEND?
Time: 15 minutes

This practice from Neff can boost our self-compassion by highlighting the difference between how we treat ourselves when we're struggling and how we treat others.[23]

1. First, think about times when a close friend feels really bad about themselves or is really struggling in some way. How do you respond to your friend in these situations (if you're at your best)?

Write down what you typically do and say, and note the tone in which you talk to your friend.

How I respond to my friend:
_____
_____
_____
_____
_____

2. Now, think about times when you feel bad about yourself or are struggling. How do you typically respond to yourself in these situations? Write down what you typically do and say, and note the tone in which you talk to yourself.

How I respond to myself:
_____
_____
_____
_____
_____

3. Did you notice a difference? If so, ask yourself why.

What factors or fears come into play that lead you to treat yourself and others so differently?

4. How do you think things might change if you responded to yourself when you're suffering in the same way you typically respond to a close friend?

How would it feel to be more compassionate toward yourself?

5. Next time you are struggling with something, try treating yourself like a good friend and see what happens.

PUTTING SELF-COMPASSION INTO PRACTICE

If you have a long history of criticizing and judging yourself, self-compassion may feel awkward and foreign at first—and habits can be hard to change. "We can't become more self-compassionate overnight. It's a practice that takes time," says Christopher Germer, a clinical psychologist who codeveloped the Mindful Self-Compassion program with Neff.[24]

In addition to the formal practices on previous pages, a simple place to start is just to notice suffering in yourself whenever it comes up, even if it's passing or minor—like a niggling worry about your achy back or a stranger's unkind word that stung a bit.

Therapist Tim Desmond suggests trying this type of self-talk: "You are feeling nervous right now, and that's OK. You are allowed to feel nervous and you don't have to make that feeling go away." Or "I know you feel nervous right now, and that's OK. Is there anything I could do to help you feel a little safer or more comfortable?"[25]

If this kind of loving attention feels uncomfortable, you could try thinking of yourself like your own coach.[26] Coaches are there for you when you're having a hard time; they want the best for you, and they're always on your side.

For Neff, self-compassion is ultimately about figuring out what we need in a particular moment and trying to give it to ourselves.[27] Germer likes to ask, "What do I need to feel safe? To be comforted, soothed, validated? To protect, provide for, motivate myself?"[28]

Sometimes we can give ourselves what we need with our words and attitude, and this is what the Self-Compassionate Letter and How Would You Treat a Friend? practices are for. But at other times, it feels easier or it's just more helpful to give ourselves what we need with our actions.[29]

With this in mind, the Center for Mindful Self-Compassion has a worksheet with ideas for caring for yourself physically, mentally, emotionally, relationally, and spiritually, including:

- pet your dog
- exercise
- take a warm bath
- watch a funny movie

- journal
- meet with friends
- take a walk in the woods
- pray[30]

> Do any of these ideas feel right for you? What do you need when you're struggling?
>
> _____
> _____
> _____
> _____
> _____
> _____

FIERCE SELF-COMPASSION

When we are hurt or suffering, it can help to soothe ourselves with the warmth and acceptance of tender self-compassion. But in some situations, we also need to protect ourselves: to speak up, say no, draw boundaries, or fight injustice.

In these cases, says Neff, we need *fierce* self-compassion.[31] It has the same three components as tender self-compassion—mindfulness, common humanity, and self-kindness—but they manifest in slightly different ways. In fierce self-compassion, *mindfulness* means acknowledging the harm we've experienced and recognizing what needs to change; *common humanity* allows us to see that when we stand up for ourselves, we are also standing up for others like us; and *self-kindness* translates into powerful, courageous action to protect ourselves.

What does that look like in practice? Maybe you're being taken advantage of by a coworker, your neighbor blasts music late at night, or a relative constantly tries to push their political views on you. Neff's Fierce Self-Compassion Break reflection goes like this:

- **Be mindful of the harm:** Say to yourself, "I clearly see the truth of what's happening," "This is not okay," "I should not be treated this way," or "This is unfair."
- **See your common humanity:** Think, "I am not alone; other people have experienced this, as well"; "By standing up for myself, I stand up for everyone"; "All human beings deserve just treatment"; or, simply, "Me, too."
- **Commit to being kind to yourself:** Remind yourself, "I will protect myself," "I will not yield," or "I am strong enough to take this on." For all of these, try to find phrases that feel empowering and ring true.[32]

This version of self-compassion motivates us to take action to stop harm or protect ourselves and others from it.[33] It might explain why more self-compassionate people are more empowered and resilient and cope better with stigma and bullying.[34, 35]

Different moments call for different versions of self-compassion, but ultimately the two types can work together, so we fiercely protect ourselves while at the same time feeling loving and compassionate.

Love, after all, is ultimately at the heart of self-compassion. Germer even says that if we practice self-compassion just to make the bad feelings go away, it will fail. "People need to be guided into practicing for its own sake, as we might care for a child with the flu, not to drive out the flu but as a simple expression of sympathy and kindness," he says. We care for ourselves because we are deserving of care.

If we practice enough, we might get to a place where all the intellectual exercises and words sink in and we meet our own pain with an instinctive wave of compassion that is just like the compassion we feel for others.

"We practice self-kindness regularly so that one day when your heart breaks, the kindness will flow naturally. And that's exactly when you need it most," says Germer.

Chapter 9
Emotion Regulation

When Sulyman Qardash was 17 years old, he had a vision: He would start Afghanistan's first post-Taliban rock band. Qardash had grown up as a refugee in Uzbekistan, and had recently moved back to his hometown of Kabul after the start of the U.S. war in Afghanistan. In 2008, he found some bandmates and formed Kabul Dreams.

The band immediately started getting death threats, but that didn't stop them from playing concerts. One day, Qardash suggested they perform a free show on a busy Kabul street corner that had recently been the site of many bombings.

"We were scared, but we went there," says Qardash. "We set up our musical instruments on the street and played—just to give some kind of hope or positive energy to that part of the neighborhood. And people really liked it."

Kabul Dreams's popularity grew, eventually taking them to the famous SXSW event in Austin, Texas. A couple of years later, the band moved to the Bay Area in California. Qardash fell in love and got married.

His perseverance and resilience helped him fulfill his dreams. But it didn't prepare him for the biggest loss of his life—their experience of a miscarriage.

After it happened, Qardash threw himself into caring for his wife, but he was unable to navigate his own deep sadness and anger. So he tried an Expressive Writing practice, where you write freely about your true feelings and thoughts about an experience of hurt for about 20 minutes straight. Qardash shared his writing experience on our *Science of Happiness* podcast.

"Back in Kabul, I used to write about my day sometimes," says Qardash. "Things like, 'On this day, an explosion happened, and then we didn't go to work or school.' But it was more informative, not about how I felt about it. Not my reaction to it. I wasn't taught like that."

Qardash had lived through war, displacement, and death threats, and now, with the Expressive Writing practice, he was ready to face his next challenge: processing his own difficult emotions.

"The reason I chose to do [the Expressive Writing practice] is that I've never done one," says Qardash. "[I'm not used to] writing about myself or about somebody that I really love. I really had to go deep down into my feelings [to know] what exactly I want to write. And it was a real encouraging process."

THE BENEFITS OF WORKING WITH UNPLEASANT EMOTIONS

When we go through hard times, we can get lost in waves of difficult feelings, becoming distracted and distant from others. While it's natural to feel sad, worried, angry, or stressed, if we get trapped in rumination or cycles of despair or anxiety, we may have trouble seeing our way out.

That's where learning skills for managing difficult feelings—what researchers call *emotion regulation*—can help us to cope better with whatever is distressing us.

Instead of assuming there's nothing we can do, we can purposefully explore our feelings—where they're coming from, what they're telling us, and what to do about them—in a way that's healthy and helpful. Rather than sitting with regret, recrimination, anxiety, or sadness, we can acknowledge the importance of our feelings, gain perspective on them, and soothe ourselves, preventing our feelings from overwhelming us.

EMOTION SUPPRESSION ISN'T THE ANSWER

Scientists understand that feelings aren't bad or good, per se; they're instructive.[1] While emotions may get a bad rap in some cases—pitted against reason or considered a sign of weakness—it's clear that they are important for our survival, helping us understand our needs in any given situation and what to do about them.

Unpleasant emotions can be clues to our deepest values and the ways we may have gotten off track. Loneliness reminds us to make time for our relationships, and anxiety might mean we've taken on too many projects. Once we've identified these inconsistencies, we can make small course corrections to point us in the right direction: setting up a weekly dinner with friends, perhaps, or deciding to say no to extra commitments in the near future. We can cope better with what is ailing us.

When we recognize that our feelings are generally beneficial, it helps us manage stressors better and helps prevent us from feeling depressed and anxious.[2] Accepting our difficult feelings as they are tends to lead us to experience fewer of them, which can benefit our mental health.[3] In contrast, *not* accepting our feelings—and, instead, judging ourselves for feeling badly—can compound our suffering and lead to depression.[4]

That's why it's important to face our emotions and not turn away from them. Counterintuitively, allowing ourselves to be sad or anxious could actually help protect us from full-blown depression and anxiety disorders.[5,6] "If we want to live more fully and be our most authentic selves, we need to turn towards our pain, not try to suppress it," says psychologist Beth Kurland.

The way we view emotions can actually affect us physically, too. When we see the benefits of stress, we show a healthier stress response in our bodies—which can help us overcome challenges.[7] "When we focus on the benefits of stress, we feel less stress about stress, pay attention to positive cues rather than threatening cues, and approach situations more confidently rather than avoid them," writes health psychologist Elissa Epel in her book *The Stress Prescription*.[8]

Finally, it just helps to believe in our own capacity to work with emotions. When we recognize that we can get better at changing problematic feelings using effective strategies, this, too, protects our mental health.[9]

THE BENEFITS OF HEALTHY EMOTION REGULATION

Not all strategies are created equal when it comes to working through difficult feelings. Drinking alcohol to numb emotion or distracting ourselves by overworking, for example, are unlikely to help in the long term, even if they provide temporary relief. Alternatively, blaming others for our feelings and lashing out at them could worsen our relationships without resolving underlying pain or anger.[10]

Instead, we need to focus on *adaptive* or healthy ways for coping with difficult feelings: to face them, understand them, and take appropriate action. People who use adaptive coping and show emotional intelligence—an understanding and appreciation of their own and others' feelings, as well as skills for regulating them—tend to have greater well-being and resilience.[11,12,13] Adaptive coping can involve many things, which we'll explore later in this chapter: gaining perspective on a situation, reframing difficulties in a more positive light, getting support from others, and more.[14,15,16,17,18]

"We've done a lot of studies which show that emotional intelligence is predictive of really important life outcomes," says Marc Brackett, founder of an emotion skills-building program called RULER. "People with higher emotional intelligence tend to have greater psychological health, are less anxious and less depressed or less burned out at work. They tend to make better decisions in life."[19]

But we can cultivate greater emotional intelligence. Finding ways to let go of rumination and cycles of negativity can help us move forward from adversity, allowing us to create more meaning and happiness in our lives. Read on to find out how to cope better with difficult feelings in your own life.

HOW WELL DO YOU REGULATE EMOTIONS?

Before we offer you emotion regulation practices to try out, we'd like to give you the opportunity to reflect on your own emotion regulation skills.[20] If you'd like, you can revisit these questions later to see if taking steps to work with unpleasant emotions made a difference.

	Strongly disagree	Disagree	Neutral	Agree	Strongly agree
I have my emotions well under control.	1	2	3	4	5
There is nothing wrong with feeling very emotional.	1	2	3	4	5
I can avoid getting upset by taking a different perspective on things.	1	2	3	4	5
It's okay if people see me being upset.	1	2	3	4	5
I am able to let go of my feelings.	1	2	3	4	5
It's okay to feel difficult emotions at times.	1	2	3	4	5
I can calm down very quickly.	1	2	3	4	5
I can tolerate being upset.	1	2	3	4	5
I know exactly what to do to get myself into a better mood.	1	2	3	4	5
I can tolerate having strong emotions.	1	2	3	4	5

Quick scoring guide: 10–30 = Low; 31–40 = Medium; 41–50 = High

EMOTION REGULATION PRACTICES

PRACTICE #1: EXPRESSIVE WRITING

Time: 15 minutes

In this practice from researcher James W. Pennebaker, you write freely about your true feelings and thoughts about an experience of hurt that has been emotionally challenging for you. Research suggests Expressive Writing can help us respond better to stress in the future, ease symptoms of post-traumatic stress disorder, and help our physical health.[21, 22, 23, 24, 25, 26]

Here's how to start:

1. **Find a comfortable time and place where you are unlikely to be disturbed.** If a private space is not available, you can tell others you need a little time to yourself.

2. **Use any writing materials that are available to you.** You can use a computer or smartphone or a physical notebook or piece of paper.

3. **Choose an experience of hurt to write about that is important to you.** Choose an event or situation you feel you can handle now—that is, don't write about a severe trauma too soon after it happened or if it feels too overwhelming.

4. **In your writing, explore what's been happening in connection to that hurtful experience, how it has affected you, and how it connects to different parts of your life.** You might tie this experience to your childhood, your relationship with your parents, people you have loved or love now, or your career.

5. **As you write about your experience, really let go and write freely whatever comes to your mind.** Don't worry about spelling or grammar.

6. **Try not to edit or judge what you write.** Remember that your writing is for your eyes only and that you are doing this for your own well-being.

7. **To the best of your ability, write without stopping for at least 20 minutes.** Do whatever you need to help you stay on task—you might listen to music, wear noise-canceling headphones, and put away distractions.

It's natural to slip into rumination or self-criticism as you write about a difficult experience, which might explain why not all studies find benefits for Expressive Writing. For that reason, try to follow the guidance above and aim to keep an open and curious attitude toward your feelings.

It's also possible that the benefits of this practice may take time to show up.[27] Writing and revisiting memories about something difficult can be painful, so don't be surprised if you initially feel activated. It might help to do a few writing sessions, spaced out a few days, that allow new insights and more acceptance to emerge.[28]

PRACTICE #2: GAINING PERSPECTIVE ON NEGATIVE EVENTS

Time: 5 minutes

This practice, based on research by Ozlem Ayduk and her colleagues, is a form of *self-distancing*, a way of looking at yourself as an observer. Research suggests it might help boost your positive emotions after a difficult event and allow unpleasant feelings to pass more quickly as compared to when you're more immersed in your feelings.[29,30]

Practice self-distancing by following these steps:

1. Take a few moments to bring to mind a difficult experience you are dealing with: some event in the past that made you sad or angry, for example, or some anxiety or worry you have about the future.

2. Try to understand your feelings using "you," "he/she/they," and "[your own name]" as much as possible. If your name is Jorge, for example, you would ask yourself, "Why does Jorge feel this way? What are the underlying causes and reasons for his feelings?" If you begin to see the event in your mind, try to watch through the eyes of a distanced, third-party observer, rather than through your own eyes.

3. The goal here is not to avoid or separate from your feelings, but to analyze them from a clearer and more helpful vantage point. Spend 3 minutes reflecting in this way, writing down your thoughts if you feel so inclined.

Although it may feel silly or strange to talk to yourself in the third person, research suggests that it can help you confront difficult feelings without becoming overwhelmed by them. Eventually, you might be able to use this kind of self-talk during difficult events as they're unfolding, such as a stressful task at work or a particularly challenging social situation.

PUTTING EMOTION REGULATION INTO PRACTICE

There are many approaches to managing challenging emotions, some of which we've covered in previous chapters.[31] Mindfulness can help us tune into our experience with an accepting attitude, creating more equanimity and reducing our stress.[32] Self-compassion can help us soothe ourselves while providing clarity during trying times.[33] Connecting with others can make us feel less alone, and practicing gratitude can help us shift from ruminating on the bad toward paying attention to the good.[34]

Here are some other strategies for working with difficult emotions and how you might go about practicing them.

Start by simply naming your feelings. Are you frustrated, hopeless, ashamed, envious? Psychologist Kurland suggests saying something like "I am feeling hurt *in this moment*," a reminder that feelings are temporary. Research suggests that labeling our emotions can reduce their intensity.[35]

Try to take an open, welcoming, or accepting attitude. Certain emotions can be uncomfortable, and it's natural to want to push them away. It will take lots of practice to do the opposite: to just allow them to be. Many experts use the metaphor of an unwanted house guest, someone you can welcome into your space without being glad they knocked on the door.

Kurland tried this herself when she was agonizing over a decision about her son's medical condition. "In a particular moment standing in the kitchen, gripped with fear and indecision, I did something that felt counterintuitive. I turned toward my fear to take a curious and closer look at what was actually there," she recalls.[36] As she did so, she felt the fear morph into the true sadness and grief that was underneath.

Do something soothing for yourself if the feelings are intense. Often this might be something physical, starting with noticing where the feelings are showing up in your body. Then, there are different ways you can soothe yourself: deep breathing or taking longer exhales; movement that you enjoy, such as walking or exercise; or physical touch in the form of a hug from a loved one or a caring hand over your own heart.

See what you can learn. With curiosity, we can try to find out where a feeling is coming from and what it might have to teach us. Kurland suggests asking yourself:

- If this feeling or part of me could talk, what might it say?
- What might it want or need?[37]

For her, the lesson was a vulnerable truth: that she couldn't fully protect her son, no matter how hard she tried. "When I peered at what lay behind that fear, I found acceptance—of life as it is, with fear being only a part of that, held in a vast expanse of love and care, for my son, and for my own human struggles," she writes.

Get some distance by imagining the future. Gaining Perspective on Negative Events helps you get distance from your troubles by taking a third-party perspective. Another way is to distance yourself in time and imagine how you would feel about the current situation in a week or a few years.[38] Often, this dials down the intensity of what we're feeling now by putting it into a broader context. In 5 years, you might barely remember the tense dispute you're having with your neighbor that's currently keeping you up at night.

Share your troubles with others, rather than keeping them to yourself. It's not always easy to ask for support. We might judge ourselves if we can't deal with our problems alone or feel we're annoying our friends. But emotion regulation, which we often think of as a solo, introspective task, is actually very social. Research suggests that our romantic partners sometimes know better than we do what we need to cheer up. And allowing others to help us navigate our emotions actually serves as practice for them to regulate their own.[39]

This is the idea behind psychotherapy, when a trained professional can listen to our problems and help us move forward. But even sharing our troubles with a friend can help us recover from stressors, especially if the friend can provide some perspective and not just encourage us to vent.[40, 41] To ensure you're not just ruminating alongside a friend, you could deliberately ask them for their advice about your situation.

"We should lean into social support during negative experiences, since our friends are sometimes a lot better at regulating our emotions than we are at regulating them ourselves," says postdoctoral researcher Razia Sahi.

Cultivate forgiveness. If you're continually experiencing anger and hurt from some harm that was done to you, forgiveness can be a powerful practice—when you are ready.

A good place to start is to clearly acknowledge to yourself what happened, including how it feels and how it's affecting your life right now. Then, you make a commitment to forgive, which means letting go of resentment and ill will. If it makes sense within your culture, you could see this as a practice *for yourself*; forgiveness doesn't have to mean letting the offender off the hook or even reconciling with them.

Ultimately, you can try to find a positive opportunity for growth in the experience: Perhaps it alerted you to something you need, which you may have to look for elsewhere, or perhaps you can now understand other people's suffering better.

Of course, forgiveness takes time; it's not a practice for an afternoon. But it's a pathway to consider if we feel hijacked by pain from the past. You can find more in-depth forgiveness practices at ggia.berkeley.edu.

Look on the bright side. Once you've explored the dark side of an experience, you might choose to contemplate some of its upsides. This isn't meant to dismiss the difficulty you're going through, so it's also something to try when you feel ready or to notice if it happens naturally.

Can you think of a positive thing about an upsetting experience, however small? You might reflect on how fighting with a friend brought some important issues out into the open and allowed you to learn something about their point of view.

Remind yourself of the value of unpleasant emotions. A simple way to get more comfortable with difficult emotions is to journal about a meaningful time when it was important for you to focus on feeling bad.[42] Perhaps you made a mistake and had to apologize and fix it, or you sat with a friend who was grieving.

Hunt out positive emotions. Pain and pleasure, difficulty and joy, can coexist. When we're struggling, small moments of positive feelings can help us endure. Researcher Lucy Hone stumbled upon this strategy after her 12-year-old daughter was killed in a car crash.[43] "I knew I had to somehow continue to top up our positive-emotion piggy banks," she says, continuing:

> *[I] very deliberately worked out ways to bring more hope, love, humor, pride, inspiration, serenity, and awe into our lives. I asked friends to accompany me on day-long walks that would draw me out of the cluttered world of the city and reconnect me with nature. Standing amid towering mountain peaks returned a measure of serenity and filled me with awe. Making myself feel small and insignificant somehow fueled my belief that we could fight this battle and would emerge out the other side. I sought*

> *out movies that would inspire me, listened to the Desert Island Discs podcast to fill me with hope, and watched my boys play music and sports to give me a sense of pride.*

Five years later, she learned from her experience that "it's possible to continue to live, laugh, and love, even while we grieve," she says. "There really is much we can do to help ourselves, and those we love, navigate life's darkest days."

We all have our dark days; even the happiest life won't be free of them. The point of emotion regulation skills is not to never feel bad, but to avoid adding suffering upon our suffering—to find ways to work with our emotions instead of fight them.

When Qardash did the Expressive Writing practice to help process the pain of his wife's miscarriage, it was extremely difficult at first. "It's not like Facebook, where you're always posting good things," says Qardash. "You would never write something like this [on social media]. It's hard."

He stared blankly at the paper for a long time, wondering what he could write to truly express his emotions over the miscarriage. He got up, made some tea, and then went back to the piece of paper. Eventually the words began to flow, and he was able to express his feelings through his writing.

"I wrote about how it makes me extremely angry to feel helpless," says Qardash. "It's like you want something really bad, something that you've been dreaming about, but deep down you know that it's out of your control. It's not like being a grade-A student or graduating from college, or passing a test."

Then Qardash's words took a different turn: He started writing about connection, his deep love for his wife, and how the silver lining was that the miscarriage brought him and his wife even closer to one another:

"I realized that at the end of the day, it's only the two of us sitting in the living room of our small apartment, caring for each other, loving and trying to make ourselves happy by making each other happy."

Eventually two turned to three: Qardash and his wife did grow their family.

And he continues to produce new music with Kabul Dreams. When things do feel dark, Qardash knows he can bring in a little light by having the courage to confront his difficult emotions.

"It took me 20-something years to actually do Expressive Writing," says Qardash. "But in the end you should do it, because you need to get over your barriers. And once you do, everything will be OK."

Chapter 10

Purpose

Selina Bilal was in a stressful place in her life. It was the end of her junior year as an undergraduate student at UC Berkeley, and she was preparing for her final exams. As a psychology major, she knew she wanted to bring about positive change for the world, but she was unsure about how.

While visiting family in her hometown of Faisalabad, Pakistan, Bilal did a little project of the imagination for our *Science of Happiness* podcast. She thought about her greater purpose in life, and how she could help achieve that purpose, through a research-backed practice called Magic Wand. She reflected on these questions:

Imagine you've been given a magic wand, and you can change anything you want to change in the world—what would you want to be different? Is there anything you can do to help move the world closer to this ideal?

Her mind painted a picture of a world that was compassionate and full of empathy. One where strangers gave each other warm smiles, and there was a balance in society between nurturing oneself and the community at large. "I want it to be warm and loving, and I want it to be trusting," Bilal says. "In this world, we're not hesitant to say, 'I love you.'"

But that wasn't exactly the environment in which Bilal grew up. She was an only child to a single mom, and there weren't many expressions of emotion in her home. After her parents divorced, Bilal went through some rough years when she wasn't able to communicate very well.

"My defense mechanism became shutting down," says Bilal. "I would just get numb and not express any love. We're not the most open family. We're very different in terms of beliefs, values, who we are." Bilal always clashed with her more conservative relatives, and felt they were cold, unavailable, and unwelcoming.

After doing the Magic Wand exercise for herself in Pakistan, Bilal was curious enough to ask her relatives what they would do if they had a Magic Wand—even though she had her doubts.

"I thought that their purpose is really different [from mine]," says Bilal. "That these are going to be such awkward conversations. Because of these differences, the thought of being vulnerable with them, talking about their purpose, was scary to me."

But when she did speak with her family and listen to them, she realized she was wrong. They, too, wanted to see a world that was more loving and compassionate. Her mom imagined an ideal world with less poverty. Her father talked about people having stronger relationships. Each relative she spoke with wanted the greater good for all, and talked about ways they could be agents for positive change in the world.

That's when it dawned on Bilal that, if she wanted to live in a more compassionate world, she needed to become a more compassionate person—starting with her own family in Pakistan. Says Bilal:

> *My purpose is compassion . . . . And yet I was selective with my compassion. I was labeling my family members, without compassion. All along, I never actually applied my own purpose to my hometown. I forgot to be open, I forgot to build bridges. So, basically, thinking about what I want the world to be got me thinking about who I want to be. And, as they say, be the change you want to see in the world.*

THE BENEFITS OF PURPOSE

Many of us have goals for ourselves, both large and small. But cultivating a sense of purpose implies a bit more than simply setting a goal. Purpose involves having a goal in life that you care deeply about and that contributes to the world beyond yourself in some productive sense. It's more akin to a life mission than an attempt at self-improvement.

We may decide to learn Spanish or play the piano proficiently, which are worthy goals but not a purpose, per se. However, if our intention in learning Spanish is to work assisting new immigrants, or if we're learning the piano to offer music lessons to underserved youth, these goals could be tied to a deeper sense of purpose.

Our purpose may include lofty ideals, like ending hunger, curing cancer, or advocating for universal health care. Or it may involve something like raising compassionate kids, planting urban gardens, or improving our office social climate. When we become clear on what changes we want to see around us and figure out how to contribute our talents and passions to achieving them, the sense of purpose it brings can carry us through life with more energy, focus, and joy.

HOW PURPOSE CONTRIBUTES TO WELL-BEING

Our purpose isn't necessarily singular, nor set for life; it can change as we grow and develop, taking on a new flavor and focus at different times.[1] However, a sense of purpose often begins in adolescence or early adulthood, a time of life when we're typically forming our personal identities, recognizing our values and strengths, and becoming more aware of world concerns. When that inner and outer focus leads to a sense of purpose, it can change the course of our life in powerful ways.

Research finds that teens who have a sense of purpose seem to exhibit other positive qualities, such as gratitude, compassion, and perseverance.[2] When researchers looked at how racially diverse teens experience purpose in everyday life, they found that teens with a stronger sense of purpose felt better and more satisfied with life.[3] Teens with purpose may be less prone to depression, which suggests purpose could protect their mental health.[4]

College students with a strong sense of purpose are more likely to rate themselves as persistent in the face of challenges, which helps them complete college.[5, 6] And college students with a purpose around helping others and contributing to society—as opposed to goals around creativity, money, or personal recognition—have greater integrity, personal growth, and generativity (a commitment to helping the next generation) 13 years later.[7]

A sense of purpose can be beneficial at any time in life—not just when you're young. One study found that teens and adults in the Midwest United States with a sense of purpose were more satisfied with life at every stage of life.[8] Having a purpose helps people see their lives as less stressful, no matter their level of distress or age.[9] And people with a sense of purpose are less likely to become depressed or anxious too.[10]

For adults in midlife, pursuing a purpose with prosocial goals is particularly effective at boosting their well-being—more so than other kinds of purpose.[11]

GOOD FOR THE MIND, GOOD FOR THE BODY

Having a purpose in life may also help protect our physical health. Research has found that older adults with a strong sense of purpose experience less disability and depression, better cognitive processing, and even greater longevity.[12, 13] One meta-analysis of many studies found that people with a purpose in life at one point in time were less likely to develop dementia up to 17 years later—even after accounting for things like their mood, activity level, age, gender, and education.[14]

In one surprising study, middle-aged and older U.S. adults suffering from heart disease had a 27% decreased risk of heart attack over 2 years if they had a strong sense of purpose.[15] Another group of purposeful older adults in the United States were 22% less likely to have a stroke within 4 years.[16]

Eric Kim of Harvard's School of Public Health, who conducted those studies—ironically, as an initial skeptic—says, "It's very interesting to see how this construct of purpose—which has long been discussed by philosophers and theologians—is associated with all of these benefits. It's not counterintuitive to me anymore."

As researcher Patrick Hill found, people who have purpose in life tend to live longer than others their age. When he analyzed data from a large group of U.S. adults aged 20 to 75, he found those reporting a stronger sense of purpose than others were 15% less likely to die over the next 14 years.[17]

Why would this be? Perhaps it's because having a sense of purpose helps us sleep better at night, and sleep is so important to health.[18] Or maybe it's because purposeful people tend to have improved cognitive fitness and retain their healthy habits, like exercising or teeth flossing.[19, 20] One study found that, during the COVID-19 pandemic, older people with a strong sense of purpose in life were less lonely and took more protective measures to avoid COVID-19.[21] Having a sense of purpose may make you both feel healthier *and* incentivize you to stay healthy.

"Perhaps because people with purpose have an overall outlook regarding the importance of their goals in life, they take care of themselves better," Kim says.

Since purpose involves a commitment to bettering the world, following your purpose path may end up helping those around you—in small and large ways. While finding your purpose isn't always effortless or straightforward, you can get started by thinking more about your life and what matters to you most. Read on to find out how.

HOW STRONG IS YOUR SENSE OF PURPOSE?

Before we offer you purpose practices to try out, we'd like to give you the opportunity to reflect on your own sense of purpose.[22] If you'd like, you can revisit these questions later to see if taking steps to cultivate purpose made a difference.

	Strongly disagree	Disagree	Neutral	Agree	Strongly agree
Most of what I do seems trivial and unimportant to me.	5	4	3	2	1
I know how I can use my talents to make a meaningful contribution to the larger world.	1	2	3	4	5
I understand what gives my life meaning and makes it feel worthwhile.	1	2	3	4	5
I put a good amount of effort into making my goals a reality.	1	2	3	4	5
I often learn something new so that I can help others.	1	2	3	4	5
I hope to leave the world better than I found it.	1	2	3	4	5
I'm excited about carrying out the plans that I set for myself.	1	2	3	4	5
I hope that the work that I do positively influences others.	1	2	3	4	5
A good portion of my daily activities move me closer to my long-term aims.	1	2	3	4	5
I volunteer to contribute to the welfare of others.	1	2	3	4	5

Quick scoring guide: 10–30 = Low; 31–40 = Medium; 41–50 = High

PURPOSE PRACTICES

PRACTICE #1: LIFE CRAFTING
Time: 1 hour

The Life Crafting practice is a way to better define your goals in life and chart a path to achieving them.[23] While honing your sense of purpose can feel daunting, this practice breaks it down into a series of short writing prompts.

1. **Identify your deepest values and passions—what's most important to you.** Below, write a list of your greatest values and what you most like to do in life. If you need help, you can think about the qualities you admire in others, skills you would like to build, or personal habits you both like and dislike.

The list of potential values is long, but as a place to start, you might reflect on which areas of life you care most about:

- Family
- Romantic relationships
- Parenting
- Friends/social life
- Work
- Education/training
- Recreation/fun
- Spirituality
- Citizenship/community life
- Physical self-care (diet, exercise, sleep)[24]

Then, you could dig deeper into specific things you value, like the following:

- Thinking up new ideas and being creative
- For everyone to be treated equally

- Being secure and safe
- Being a good person
- Listening to people who are different from you
- Being humble and modest
- Having fun
- Being independent
- Helping others
- Adventure and excitement
- Caring for the environment[25]

Then, you can reflect on what you're passionate about in life—whether that's music or art, technology, sports, or travel.

My passions and values:
_____
_____
_____
_____
_____
_____
_____
_____

2. **Reflect on your ideal future.** Write a paragraph envisioning how you'd like your social life or your career path to turn out at some future age—like 10 or 20 years down the road—if you had no constraints. What does your life look like? What kinds of personal and professional relationships do you have? What is your job or volunteer role? What is important to you? What do you really care about, and why?

In my ideal future . . .

3. **Write down how you'll attain your goals.** Based on this ideal future life that you imagine, prioritize some goals that could help you get there. Separately, identify obstacles in the way of those goals, and describe your strategy for overcoming them.

Potential goals to work on:

Some obstacles I might encounter and how to deal with them:

5. **Make a public commitment to your goals.** Communicate these goals to others in your community, including friends, family, and coworkers.

PRACTICE #2: MAGIC WAND

Time: 15 minutes

This writing activity, from Kendall Cotton Bronk and her colleagues, offers one way to reflect on your purpose that could reveal some new ideas and opportunities. Research suggests that, along with other purpose practices, it can help people feel more successful at searching for and identifying a purpose in life.[26]

To start, think about the world in which you live. This includes your home, your community, and the world at large.

Imagine you've been given a magic wand, and you can change anything you want to change in the world. What would you want to be different? Why?

In my ideal world . . .

_____
_____
_____
_____

Now, reflect on what it would take to change the world in this way. Is there anything you can do to help move the world closer to this ideal? If so, explain how; if not, explain why not.

You can be as creative and imaginative as you want for this practice. Use whatever writing style you like, and do not worry about spelling or grammar.

How can I make this world a reality?
_____
_____
_____
_____
_____
_____
_____
_____

PUTTING PURPOSE INTO PRACTICE

Before we offer some more tips for deepening your sense of purpose, let's clear up a few misconceptions to help ease any worries or frustrations you might have.

First, unlike some of the other skills in this workbook, purpose isn't something you can cultivate in a 10-minute practice. According to developmental psychologist and purpose researcher Kendall Bronk, most people find purpose in a meandering way—through a combination of education, experience, and self-reflection, often helped along by encouragement from others.[27] That means that you may naturally develop a sense of purpose over time, but you can also take deliberate steps to help that process along.

In other good news, we don't have to worry about finding our *one true purpose*; we can find purpose in different areas of life. In the family realm, we may find a deep sense of purpose from being a loving aunt or taking care of aging parents. At work, we might feel fulfilled in supporting our coworkers, making a difference in the organization, or contributing to society, suggests William Damon, a purpose researcher and director of the Stanford Center on Adolescence.[28]

Also, it's normal for our sense of purpose to wax and wane throughout life and for us to go through stages when we're searching for a renewed purpose. During life transitions, we might find ourselves at a crossroads, when one purpose (e.g., raising kids) moves to the back burner and we're looking for a new focus.

With all that in mind, here are a few ideas to get you started thinking about purpose. Hopefully, some of them will spark insights for you that can lead to further exploration.

REFLECT ON YOURSELF, YOUR LIFE, AND THE WORLD

In addition to your values and passions, which we explored in the Life Crafting practice, another good place to start is to think about your strengths. It feels meaningful when we're able to apply what we're good at to something we care about.

What are your unique strengths? Some of them could be strengths of character; perhaps you exhibit bravery, fairness, humility, leadership, open-mindedness, patience, gratitude, or service to others.[29] Or maybe you have specific skills and talents that you excel at, like an easygoing way with people, an ability to simplify complex ideas, or an aptitude for machines and computers.

My strengths:

_____
_____
_____
_____
_____
_____

Other inspiration might come from our past. It's common for our purpose to grow out of difficult experiences we went through or witnessed others go through.[30]

Mariah Jordan from Cleveland, one of the winners of the GGSC Purpose Challenge Scholarship Contest, often accompanied her grandmother to doctors' appointments as a child. Over time, witnessing her grandmother's experiences, she began to see the racial inequalities that existed in health care. She went on to volunteer in a medical setting and conduct research on cancer in African Americans, working to eliminate health disparities and bring more cultural sensitivity to the field of medicine.[31]

You might even think about your strengths in this context: What obstacles have you encountered? What strengths helped you overcome them? How did your strengths help make life better for others?

If you find it hard to answer these questions about yourself, you could ask for feedback from people who know you—like teachers, friends, family, colleagues, and mentors. They might have a helpful perspective on what you're good at, what you seem to like to do, and how you might make your mark on the world.

Finally, think about the people you admire. Reading about the work of civil rights leaders or activists can be uplifting and motivate us to work toward the greater good.[32] However, sometimes hearing about these larger-than-life examples can be intimidating.[33] If so, you can look to everyday people who are doing good in smaller ways. Maybe you have a friend who volunteers to collect food for the homeless or a colleague whose work in promoting liberty inspires you.

TRY OUT NEW THINGS

Finding purpose involves more than just self-reflection. According to Bronk, purpose is about trying new things and seeing how those activities enable you to use your skills to make a meaningful difference in the world.

Because purpose involves serving the broader world, it's natural to be lacking in purpose if we're isolated. That's why finding a community you feel connected to can help.

"If you're having trouble remembering your purpose, take a look at the people around you. What do you have in common with them? What are they trying to be? What impact do you see them having on the world? Is that impact a positive one? Can you join with them in making that impact? What do they need? Can you give it to them?" writes the GGSC's Jeremy Adam Smith.[34]

Volunteering with a community organization focused on something of interest to you could put you in touch with people who have similar values, who may inspire you or suggest other opportunities for making a difference that you hadn't thought of before.

Gary Maxworthy was 56 when his wife died from cancer. After more than three decades in food distribution, he wanted to give back. He started volunteering at a food bank, where he quickly noticed a big problem and a big opportunity: Growers were having to send lots of imperfect produce to landfills, because they couldn't sell it, and accepting fresh produce was too difficult for food banks. He created Farm to Family to solve that problem and ensure that fresh fruit and vegetables make it to families in need.[35]

One kind of connection that can be particularly powerful is when you spend time with people of different ages than you. Younger people can find guidance from mentors and role models, whereas older people can find purpose in passing on life experiences to others.[36, 37]

"Mama" Vy Higginsen is the founder of the Mama Foundation for the Arts, which aims to uplift Black music and help people heal through making music together. In the process, she's sharing the music of older generations with teens and young people, some of whom go on to become performing artists or activists.[38]

BE PATIENT

Deep down, Bronk believes that everyone has a purpose, even if they don't realize it or know what it is yet.

"We all have things that we care about, we all have special talents that we can apply to make a meaningful difference in the world around us," she says. Other researchers agree that you can have a sense of purpose even if you can't write it down in a simple sentence: "My purpose is . . . "

Sometimes, it may seem that other people have it all figured out, and we're the only ones floundering. But it's normal for our purpose journey to take time. Being patient will make that process more enjoyable and help us weather the ebbs and flows of purposefulness that naturally happen across our lives. Ultimately, purpose is a constant practice of orienting ourselves toward what matters to us and asking, as one nonprofit CEO does, *how can I be useful*?[39]

For Selina Bilal, her purpose was to help build a more compassionate world. After doing the Magic Wand practice with her family in Pakistan, she realized that compassion had to start with herself. She needed to open her ears and heart to all people around her, not just those with whom she agreed.

"When I actually started talking with my family about the greater good, it turned out to bring us together," says Bilal. "We ended up sharing our own vulnerabilities with each other, which made me realize we're not all that different. Yes, there are differences, but we tend to accentuate them so much more than our similarities. At the end of the day, we're pretty much the same."

This understanding furthered Bilal's own purpose in life. In addition to cultivating a more compassionate world, she believed people also needed to build bridges. She imagined a world in which we truly listen to others' perspectives, considering who they are and why they became the way they are and treating them with empathy and compassion. Where we learn from each other's differences, rather than letting them drive us apart.

In line with the research, doing the Magic Wand practice helped Bilal in her purpose journey. She felt more hopeful, optimistic, and motivated to truly be a force of compassion in the world.

"I feel like this [Magic Wand] activity really helped me think deeper about my purpose, and think about my goals and what they mean to me. It was really impactful in helping me realize my own purpose in life."

● CONCLUSION

At the start of this workbook, we said that happiness is not something you achieve, but a constant habit and practice. We hope that thinking about well-being in this way, and learning about all the skills you can cultivate, gives you a greater sense of hope and agency in your own life.

Whether you tried one practice in this book or all of them, you can wake up tomorrow and take a small step toward a new habit—maybe in the few minutes before you leave for work, on your commute, at dinner with your family, or with your children before bed.

"The key to happiness lies ... in our daily intentional activities," writes researcher Sonja Lyubomirsky in her book *The How of Happiness*. "[You] can influence your life from this day forward in a significant and meaningful way. This is where you can begin."[1]

MAKE YOUR HAPPINESS PLAN

If we want to change our habits, it helps to have a plan—and to predict the stumbling blocks we might encounter before they arise. To that end, we'd like to help you make a plan to continue engaging in some of the practices from this workbook. Even if you just pick one and stick with it, it could make a difference in your life.

When choosing happiness practices, researchers suggest a few considerations. In general, it's typically better to select activities that feel natural, enjoyable, or valuable to you—something you'll be able to keep up with because it comes easily to you, it's interesting or challenging in a positive way, or it aligns with your identity. It's better to steer clear of practices that you might do out of guilt or because someone else wants you to.[2]

Another consideration is how your cultural background comes into play.

Unfortunately, as in many fields, well-being research has historically been more representative of white and Western experiences. One survey of psychology research from 1974 to 2018 found that the majority of top journal editors and first authors on papers were white.[3] Many psychology studies target the easy-to-reach audience of Western college students. Not only that, but the surveys used to measure levels of well-being may also reflect Western conceptions of happiness if they were developed and tested on Western populations, skewing our understanding of who is happy and how.

What well-being means to you depends partly on your culture. Rather than getting happier individually, you may feel more motivated by practices that enhance your relationships and benefit others. Additionally, some cultures, like that of the United States, tend to place a higher emphasis on high-energy emotions like excitement, enthusiasm, and elation than certain others, which tend to prefer more low-energy emotions like calm, peacefulness, and relaxation.[4] Of course, while we're influenced by our culture, each individual has their own unique profile of emotions they seek out and others they'd rather avoid.

These considerations are helpful to keep in mind as you consider your Happiness Plan. If a practice doesn't fit with your values or cultural practices, look for ones that feel more aligned with you. And consider what emotions you'd like to cultivate in your life, whether it's the calm of a meditation or the thrill of making small talk with a stranger.

REFLECT

What does happiness mean to you?

_____

_____

YOUR HAPPINESS PLAN

Which practices have you tried so far?

- ☐ **Small Talk:** Strike up a brief conversation with a stranger.
- ☐ **Capitalizing on Positive Events:** Respond with enthusiasm to someone's good news.
- ☐ **Feeling Connected:** Journal about a time you felt particularly close to someone.
- ☐ **Random Acts of Kindness:** Perform five acts of kindness, all in one day.
- ☐ **Gift of Time:** Spend time with someone, or do something for them on your own.
- ☐ **Active Listening:** Listen attentively with the goal of understanding and empathizing.
- ☐ **Shared Identity:** Look for things you have in common with someone who seems different from you.
- ☐ **Compassion Meditation:** Extend warm, loving feelings toward yourself and others.
- ☐ **Feeling Supported:** Journal about a time when someone supported you.
- ☐ **Awe Outing:** Spend time outdoors looking for wonder and inspiration.
- ☐ **Noticing Nature:** Take photos of natural scenes that evoke emotion in you.
- ☐ **Body Scan Meditation:** Bring mindfulness to each part of your body in turn.

- ☐ **Mindful Breathing:** Focus gentle attention on your breath, without judgment.
- ☐ **Self-Compassion Letter:** Write yourself a letter expressing compassion, understanding, and acceptance of something with which you struggle.
- ☐ **How Would You Treat a Friend?:** When you're struggling, talk to yourself the way a close friend would.
- ☐ **Gratitude Letter:** Write a letter to someone you never properly thanked.
- ☐ **Gratitude Journal:** Write down the things for which you are grateful.
- ☐ **Expressive Writing:** Journal about your thoughts and feelings around an emotional challenge.
- ☐ **Gaining Perspective on Negative Events:** Take a third-person perspective on a problem in your life.
- ☐ **Life Crafting:** Reflect on your values, ideal future, and goals.
- ☐ **Magic Wand:** Identify what you'd like to change about the world.

Which practices do you want to try in the future? Go back and underline them above.

Make a plan: Pick one to three practices you want to keep working on. When, where, and how will you try these practices?

For example: I will take an Awe Outing on my way home from work on Friday.

_____

_____

_____

What obstacles might you encounter, and how could you overcome them?

For example: I'm tired at the end of the day and sometimes I don't feel like meditating. Maybe I could try listening to a meditation during my commute.

Finding the practices that work for you, and figuring out when and how often to engage in them, might take some trial and error.

One thing you want to avoid is a practice getting stale and routine over time. Counterintuitively, for example, one study found that keeping a gratitude journal once a week might be more beneficial than several times a week.[5]

Variety also helps, even if you're doing the same general practice. People who perform different acts of kindness—from taking out the trash for a roommate to loaning a friend a book—tend to get happier in a week than people who do the same act of kindness over and over.[6]

"Variety is not only the spice of life, but the spice of happiness as well," write the authors behind that research, Kennon M. Sheldon, Julia Boehm, and Lyubomirsky.

At the same time, you can also expect to see more benefits if you're able to stick with something over time, rather than just dabbling in it once or twice. So finding a balance between a commitment to a new habit and trying to keep it fun and interesting is a good goal.

If you know what new habit you'd like to adopt but you struggle to stick with it, there are a few tools at your disposal. You could start small, with something that takes less than 5 minutes to accomplish; for example, try out a short meditation rather than forcing yourself to sit in silence for 20 minutes.[7] In addition to making the activity easy at first, it also helps to make it fun and rewarding. If you recruit a friend for your Awe Outing, you'll not only have some accountability but you might also enjoy it more.

If it's hard to remember your new habit in the first place, try to tie it to a regular trigger in your life,[8] like your kids leaving for school or brushing your teeth. You can even add little reminders to your physical environment, whether that's a note on your calendar, an image on your computer desktop, or a meaningful piece of jewelry.[9]

Finally, be sure to slow down and savor how the new habit makes you feel—a little added mindfulness. Spend an extra few seconds with the warm feelings of gratitude, or awe, or connection that your new habit evokes. And remember why it's important to you to cultivate that quality in the first place.[10]

ACKNOWLEDGE WHAT YOU CAN'T CONTROL

Our happiness is shaped by individual choices, genetics, life experience, social forces, and culture. This workbook focuses on the individual choices you can make to shift your happiness, but we'd be remiss if we didn't acknowledge all those other factors.

Social and structural forces like racism and sexism, political conflict, and economic inequality affect our lives in profound ways that influence well-being.

Government policies also play a role, including laws around employee rights, working conditions, and access to health care; parental leave policies affect the happiness of parents.[11] Part of your own happiness, and the differences in happiness around the world, can be attributed to these larger forces.

As the Greater Good Science Center's Jeremy Adam Smith writes, "There are events and forces at work today that are simply making happiness much less likely for many people, and which seem to be widening 'happiness gaps' between the most privileged and everyone else."[12, 13]

Even just trying the practices in this book requires free time and a relatively safe environment, which are not accessible to everyone.

These reflections aren't meant to be discouraging, but rather a reminder to us all to offer compassion to ourselves when we're struggling, often through no fault of our own. When life is hard, it's not always the case that doing this or that practice will magically make things better—although it probably can help a little when you're ready, if you have the energy, time, and space to try.

DON'T OBSESS OVER HAPPINESS

Believing you have total control over your own happiness is counterproductive—and so is believing you can or should be happy all the time.

Happiness is a worthy aim—one that can improve your health, make the people around you happier, and maybe even help you work for social change.[14, 15, 16] But in the end, it may be better to aim for happiness indirectly, focusing on skills like gratitude and kindness and self-compassion that have been found to contribute to it, rather than putting all your focus on happiness itself.

As we've discussed several times already, it's not realistic or healthy to expect a constant stream of positive emotions. Multiple studies suggest that experiencing and embracing a range of emotions, not just the pleasant ones, is good for our mental and physical health.[17]

There's also some research to suggest that obsessing about feeling happy doesn't work. If we value happiness obsessively, we tend to feel fewer positive emotions and more unpleasant emotions and be more depressed and less satisfied with life.[18] On top of that, we tend to feel worse when we try to feel happy during an already pleasant experience or monitor our feelings moment to moment.[19, 20]

"People who strive to feel good every possible moment, as if it were possible to will oneself to be happy, appear to be following a recipe for unhappiness," says researcher Lahnna Catalino.[21] You might be falling into this trap if you believe happiness is a measure of how worthwhile your life is, you feel you should be happy all the time, and not feeling happy—even for just a day—makes you wonder if something is wrong.

Ultimately, having a judgmental attitude about our own emotional experience, and comparing it to some imagined ideal, isn't going to bring us the contentment we seek. We can certainly carve out happy moments and look for the positives in life. But it's more about focusing on the person we want to be—whether that's a purposeful parent, a kind neighbor and friend, or a resilient leader—and embracing the journey that we're on.

We are excited about the promise of the practices and research in this workbook and the new studies and experiments that are being conducted every day in laboratories across the world to help us all live more meaningful lives and build more compassionate societies. This research isn't perfect, but like all good science, it evolves over time. And there is already so much helpful guidance it can offer us.

All it takes is a small change to create a ripple effect. You can bring more connection, compassion, and meaning to your own life and to the lives of the people around you.

REFERENCES

INTRODUCTION

1. Bartels, M. (2015). Genetics of wellbeing and its components satisfaction with life, happiness, and quality of life: A review and meta-analysis of heritability studies. *Behavior Genetics*, *45*(2), 137–156. https://doi.org/10.1007/s10519-015-9713-y

CHAPTER 1

1. Martín-María, N., Caballero, F. F., Miret, M., Tyrovolas, S., Haro, J. M., Ayuso-Mateos, J. L., & Chatterji, S. (2019). Differential impact of transient and chronic loneliness on health status: A longitudinal study. *Psychology & Health*, *35*(2), 177–195. https://doi.org/10.1080/08870446.2019.1632312
2. Kross, E., Berman, M. G., Mischel, W., Smith, E. E., & Wager, T. D. (2011). Social rejection shares somatosensory representations with physical pain. *Proceedings of the National Academy of Sciences*, *108*(15), 6270–6275. https://doi.org/10.1073/pnas.1102693108
3. Uchino, B. N., Landvatter, J., Zee, K., & Bolger, N. (2020). Social support and antibody responses to vaccination: A meta-analysis. *Annals of Behavioral Medicine*, *54*(8), 567–574. https://doi.org/10.1093/abm/kaaa029
4. Walker, E., Ploubidis, G., & Fancourt, D. (2019). Social engagement and loneliness are differentially associated with neuro-immune markers in older age: Time-varying associations from the English Longitudinal Study of Ageing. *Brain Behavior and Immunity*, *82*, 224–229. https://doi.org/10.1016/j.bbi.2019.08.189
5. Valtorta, N. K., Kanaan, M., Gilbody, S., Ronzi, S., & Hanratty, B. (2016). Loneliness and social isolation as risk factors for coronary heart disease and stroke: Systematic review and meta-analysis of longitudinal observational studies. *Heart*, *102*(13), 1009–1016. https://doi.org/10.1136/heartjnl-2015-308790

6. Chida, Y., Hamer, M., Wardle, J., & Steptoe, A. (2008). Do stress-related psychosocial factors contribute to cancer incidence and survival? *Nature Clinical Practice Oncology*, *5*(8), 466–475. https://doi.org/10.1038/ncponc1134
7. Brinkhues, S., Dukers-Muijrers, N. H. T. M., Hoebe, C. J. P. A., Van Der Kallen, C. J. H., Dagnelie, P. C., Koster, A., Henry, R. M. A., Sep, S. J. S., Schaper, N. C., Stehouwer, C. D. A., Bosma, H., Savelkoul, P. H. M., & Schram, M. T. (2017). Socially isolated individuals are more prone to have newly diagnosed and prevalent type 2 diabetes mellitus - the Maastricht study -. *BMC Public Health*, *17*(1), 955. https://doi.org/10.1186/s12889-017-4948-6
8. *Welcome to the Harvard study on adult development.* (n.d.). Harvard Second Generation Study. Retrieved August 7, 2024, from https://www.adultdevelopmentstudy.org/
9. Suttie, J. (2023, February 6). What the longest happiness study reveals about finding fulfillment. *Greater Good*. https://greatergood.berkeley.edu/article/item/what_the_longest_happiness_study_reveals_about_finding_fulfillment
10. *Dunedin multidisciplinary health & development research unit.* (n.d.). University of Otago. Retrieved August 7, 2024, from https://dunedinstudy.otago.ac.nz/
11. *1970 British Cohort Study.* (n.d.) University College London Centre for Longitudinal Studies. Retrieved August 7, 2024, from https://cls.ucl.ac.uk/cls-studies/1970-british-cohort-study/
12. *Healthy Aging in Neighborhoods of Diversity Across the Life Span.* (n.d.) Retrieved August 7, 2024, from https://handls.nih.gov/
13. Card, K. G., & Skakoon-Sparling, S. (2023). Are social support, loneliness, and social connection differentially associated with happiness across levels of introversion-extraversion? *Health Psychology Open*, *10*(1). https://doi.org/10.1177/20551029231184034
14. Diener, E., & Seligman, M. E. (2002). Very happy people. *Psychological Science*, *13*(1), 81–84. https://doi.org/10.1111/1467-9280.00415
15. Rohrer, J. M., Richter, D., Brümmer, M., Wagner, G. G., & Schmukle, S. C. (2018). Successfully striving for happiness: Socially engaged pursuits predict increases in life satisfaction. *Psychological Science*, *29*(8), 1291–1298. https://doi.org/10.1177/0956797618761660
16. Kahneman, D., Krueger, A. B., Schkade, D. A., Schwarz, N., & Stone, A. A. (2004). A survey method for characterizing daily life experience: The day reconstruction method. *Science*, *306*(5702), 1776–1780. https://doi.org/10.1126/science.1103572
17. Debats, D. L. (1999). Sources of meaning: An investigation of significant commitments in life. *Journal of Humanistic Psychology*, *39*(4), 30–57. https://doi.org/10.1177/0022167899394003
18. Celidwen, Y. (2022, September 7). Why we need Indigenous wisdom. *Mind & Life Institute*. https://www.mindandlife.org/insight/why-we-need-indigenous-wisdom/
19. Suttie, J. (2013, December 2). Why are we so wired to connect? *Greater Good*. https://greatergood.berkeley.edu/article/item/why_are_we_so_wired_to_connect
20. Lieberman, M. D. (2013). *Social: Why our brains are wired to connect.* Crown.
21. Ranson, K. E., & Urichuk, L. J. (2008). The effect of parent–child attachment relationships

on child biopsychosocial outcomes: A review. *Early Child Development and Care, 178*(2), 129–152. https://doi.org/10.1080/03004430600685282

22. Bachar, E., Canetti, L., Bonne, O., De-Nour, A. K., & Shalev, A. Y. (1997). Pre-adolescent chumship as a buffer against psychopathology in adolescents with weak family support and weak parental bonding. *Child Psychiatry & Human Development, 27*(4), 209–220. https://doi.org/10.1007/bf02353350

23. Robinson, S., White, A., & Anderson, E. (2017). Privileging the bromance: A critical appraisal of romantic and bromantic relationships. *Men and Masculinities, 22*(5), 850–871. https://doi.org/10.1177/1097184x17730386

24. Olsson, C. A., McGee, R., Nada-Raja, S., & Williams, S. M. (2012). A 32-year longitudinal study of child and adolescent pathways to well-being in adulthood. *Journal of Happiness Studies, 14*(3), 1069–1083. https://doi.org/10.1007/s10902-012-9369-8

25. Cundiff, J. M., & Matthews, K. A. (2018). Friends with health benefits: The long-term benefits of early peer social integration for blood pressure and obesity in midlife. *Psychological Science, 29*(5), 814–823. https://doi.org/10.1177/0956797617746510

26. Sandstrom, G. M., & Dunn, E. W. (2014). Social interactions and well-being: The surprising power of weak ties. *Personality and Social Psychology Bulletin, 40*(7), 910–922. https://doi.org/10.1177/0146167214529799

27. Kauppi, M., Kawachi, I., Batty, G. D., Oksanen, T., Elovainio, M., Pentti, J., Aalto, V., Virtanen, M., Koskenvuo, M., Vahtera, J., & Kivimäki, M. (2017). Characteristics of social networks and mortality risk: Evidence from 2 prospective cohort studies. *American Journal of Epidemiology, 187*(4), 746–753. https://doi.org/10.1093/aje/kwx301

28. Epley, N., & Schroeder, J. (2014). Mistakenly seeking solitude. *Journal of Experimental Psychology General, 143*(5), 1980–1999. https://doi.org/10.1037/a0037323

29. Lee, R. M., Draper, M., & Lee, S. (2001). Social connectedness, dysfunctional interpersonal behaviors, and psychological distress: Testing a mediator model. *Journal of Counseling Psychology, 48*(3), 310–318. https://doi.org/10.1037/0022-0167.48.3.310

30. Gable, S. L., Gonzaga, G. C., & Strachman, A. (2006). Will you be there for me when things go right? Supportive responses to positive event disclosures. *Journal of Personality and Social Psychology, 91*(5), 904–917. https://doi.org/10.1037/0022-3514.91.5.904

31. Hovasapian, A., & Levine, L. J. (2018). Keeping the magic alive: Social sharing of positive life experiences sustains happiness. *Cognition and Emotion, 32*(8), 1559–1570. https://doi.org/10.1080/02699931.2017.1422697

32. Pavey, L., Greitemeyer, T., & Sparks, P. (2011). Highlighting relatedness promotes prosocial motives and behavior. *Personality and Social Psychology Bulletin, 37*(7), 905–917. https://doi.org/10.1177/0146167211405994

33. Newman, K. (2023, August 15). Other people may not be the solution to loneliness. *Greater Good.* https://greatergood.berkeley.edu/article/item/other_people_may_not_be_the_solution_to_loneliness

34. Stavrova, O., & Ren, D. (2023). Alone in a crowd: Is social contact associated with less psychological pain of loneliness in everyday life? *Journal of Happiness Studies, 24*(5), 1841–1860. https://doi.org/10.1007/s10902-023-00661-3
35. Masi, C. M., Chen, H., Hawkley, L. C., & Cacioppo, J. T. (2010). A meta-analysis of interventions to reduce loneliness. *Personality and Social Psychology Review, 15*(3), 219–266. https://doi.org/10.1177/1088868310377394
36. Simon, E. B., & Walker, M. P. (2018). Sleep loss causes social withdrawal and loneliness. *Nature Communications, 9*(1). https://doi.org/10.1038/s41467-018-05377-0
37. Page, R. M., & Hammermeister, J. (1995). Shyness and loneliness: Relationship to the exercise frequency of college students. *Psychological Reports, 76*(2), 395–398. https://doi.org/10.2466/pr0.1995.76.2.395
38. Lindsay, E. K., Young, S., Brown, K. W., Smyth, J. M., & Creswell, J. D. (2019). Mindfulness training reduces loneliness and increases social contact in a randomized controlled trial. *Proceedings of the National Academy of Sciences, 116*(9), 3488–3493. https://doi.org/10.1073/pnas.1813588116
39. American Psychiatric Association. (2024, January 30). *New APA poll: One in three Americans feels lonely every week*. https://www.psychiatry.org/news-room/news-releases/new-apa-poll-one-in-three-americans-feels-lonely-e
40. *The loneliness epidemic persists: A post-pandemic look at the state of loneliness among U.S. adults*. (n.d.). The Cigna Group Newsroom. https://newsroom.thecignagroup.com/loneliness-epidemic-persists-post-pandemic-look
41. Newman, K. (2023, February 21). Want better relationships? Here's what to do today. *Greater Good*. https://greatergood.berkeley.edu/article/item/want_better_relationships_heres_what_to_do_today
42. Suttie, J. (2020, November 2). Should you call or text? Science weighs in. *Greater Good*. https://greatergood.berkeley.edu/article/item/should_you_call_or_text_science_weighs_in
43. Rholes, W. S., Paetzold, R. L., & Kohn, J. L. (2016). Disorganized attachment mediates the link from early trauma to externalizing behavior in adult relationships. *Personality and Individual Differences, 90*, 61–65. https://doi.org/10.1016/j.paid.2015.10.043
44. Park, Y., Johnson, M. D., MacDonald, G., & Impett, E. A. (2019). Perceiving gratitude from a romantic partner predicts decreases in attachment anxiety. *Developmental Psychology, 55*(12), 2692–2700. https://doi.org/10.1037/dev0000830
45. Hopper, E. (2017, September 19). Can you cultivate a more secure attachment style? *Greater Good*. https://greatergood.berkeley.edu/article/item/can_you_cultivate_a_more_secure_attachment_style
46. Bruk, A., Scholl, S. G., & Bless, H. (2018). Beautiful mess effect: Self–other differences in evaluation of showing vulnerability. *Journal of Personality and Social Psychology, 115*(2), 192–205. https://doi.org/10.1037/pspa0000120

47. Collins, N. L., & Miller, L. C. (1994). Self-disclosure and liking: A meta-analytic review. *Psychological Bulletin, 116*(3), 457–475. https://doi.org/10.1037/0033-2909.116.3.457
48. Brown, B. (2010, June). *The power of vulnerability* [Video]. TED Talks. https://www.ted.com/talks/brene_brown_the_power_of_vulnerability

CHAPTER 2

1. Knudsen, J. D. (2006, March 1). Little helpers. *Greater Good.* https://greatergood.berkeley.edu/article/item/little_helpers
2. Aknin, L. B., Hamlin, J. K., & Dunn, E. W. (2012). Giving leads to happiness in young children. *PLoS ONE, 7*(6), e39211. https://doi.org/10.1371/journal.pone.0039211
3. Rossi, G., Dingemanse, M., Floyd, S., Baranova, J., Blythe, J., Kendrick, K. H., Zinken, J., & Enfield, N. J. (2023). Shared cross-cultural principles underlie human prosocial behavior at the smallest scale. *Scientific Reports, 13*(1). https://doi.org/10.1038/s41598-023-30580-5
4. Nelson, S. K., Layous, K., Cole, S. W., & Lyubomirsky, S. (2016). Do unto others or treat yourself? The effects of prosocial and self-focused behavior on psychological flourishing. *Emotion, 16*(6), 850–861. https://doi.org/10.1037/emo0000178
5. Datu, J. A. D., Wong, G. S. P., & Rubie-Davies, C. (2021). Can kindness promote media literacy skills, self-esteem, and social self-efficacy among selected female secondary school students? An intervention study. *Computers & Education, 161*, 104062. https://doi.org/10.1016/j.compedu.2020.104062
6. Yang, Y., Zhao, H., Aidi, M., & Kou, Y. (2018). Three good deeds and three blessings: The kindness and gratitude interventions with Chinese prisoners. *Criminal Behaviour and Mental Health, 28*(5), 433–441. https://doi.org/10.1002/cbm.2085
7. Dunn, E. W., Aknin, L. B., & Norton, M. I. (2014). Prosocial spending and happiness: Using money to benefit others pays off. *Current Directions in Psychological Science, 23*(1), 41–47. https://doi.org/10.1177/0963721413512503
8. Aknin, L. B., Dunn, E. W., & Whillans, A. V. (2022). The emotional rewards of prosocial spending are robust and replicable in large samples. *Current Directions in Psychological Science, 31*(6), 536–545. https://doi.org/10.1177/09637214221121100
9. Aknin, L. B., Dunn, E. W., Proulx, J., Lok, I., & Norton, M. I. (2020). Does spending money on others promote happiness?: A registered replication report. *Journal of Personality and Social Psychology, 119*(2), e15–e26. https://doi.org/10.1037/pspa0000191
10. Varma, M. M., Chen, D., Lin, X., Aknin, L. B., & Hu, X. (2023). Prosocial behavior promotes positive emotion during the COVID-19 pandemic. *Emotion, 23*(2), 538–553. https://doi.org/10.1037/emo0001077
11. Titova, L., & Sheldon, K. M. (2021). Happiness comes from trying to make others feel good, rather than oneself. *The Journal of Positive Psychology, 17*(3), 341–355. https://doi.org/10.1080/17439760.2021.1897867

12. Hui, B. P. H., Ng, J. C. K., Berzaghi, E., Cunningham-Amos, L. A., & Kogan, A. (2020). Rewards of kindness? A meta-analysis of the link between prosociality and well-being. *Psychological Bulletin, 146*(12), 1084–1116. https://doi.org/10.1037/bul0000298
13. Whillans, A. V., Dunn, E. W., Sandstrom, G. M., Dickerson, S. S., & Madden, K. M. (2016). Is spending money on others good for your heart? *Health Psychology, 35*(6), 574–583. https://doi.org/10.1037/hea0000332
14. Maran, M. (2009, June 1). The activism cure. *Greater Good.* https://greatergood.berkeley.edu/article/item/the_activism_cure/
15. Oman, D., Thoresen, C. E., & Mcmahon, K. (1999). Volunteerism and mortality among the community-dwelling elderly. *Journal of Health Psychology, 4*(3), 301–316. https://doi.org/10.1177/135910539900400301
16. Brown, S. L., Nesse, R. M., Vinokur, A. D., & Smith, D. M. (2003). Providing social support may be more beneficial than receiving it: Results from a prospective study of mortality. *Psychological Science, 14*(4), 320–327. https://doi.org/10.1111/1467-9280.14461
17. Jung, H., Seo, E., Han, E., Henderson, M. D., & Patall, E. A. (2020). Prosocial modeling: A meta-analytic review and synthesis. *Psychological Bulletin, 146*(8), 635–663. https://doi.org/10.1037/bul0000235
18. *Altruism quiz.* (2011, December). Greater Good. https://greatergood.berkeley.edu/quizzes/take_quiz/altruism
19. Gander, F., Proyer, R. T., Ruch, W., & Wyss, T. (2013). Strength-based positive interventions: Further evidence for their potential in enhancing well-being and alleviating depression. *Journal of Happiness Studies, 14*(4), 1241–1259. https://dx.doi.org/10.1007/s10902-012-9380-0
20. Suttie, J. (2022, November 7). Do you underestimate the impact of being kind? *Greater Good.* https://greatergood.berkeley.edu/article/item/do_you_underestimate_the_impact_of_being_kind
21. Boothby, E. J., & Bohns, V. K. (2020). Why a simple act of kindness is not as simple as it seems: Underestimating the positive impact of our compliments on others. *Personality and Social Psychology Bulletin, 47*(5), 826–840. https://doi.org/10.1177/0146167220949003
22. Darley, J. M., & Batson, C. D. (1973). "From Jerusalem to Jericho": A study of situational and dispositional variables in helping behavior. *Journal of Personality and Social Psychology, 27*(1), 100–108. https://doi.org/10.1037/h0034449
23. Mogilner, C., Chance, Z., & Norton, M. I. (2012). Giving time gives you time. *Psychological Science, 23*(10), 1233–1238. https://doi.org/10.1177/0956797612442551
24. Cregg, D. R., & Cheavens, J. S. (2022). Healing through helping: An experimental investigation of kindness, social activities, and reappraisal as well-being interventions. *The Journal of Positive Psychology, 18*(6), 924–941. https://doi.org/10.1080/17439760.2022.2154695
25. Svoboda, E. (2021, November 16). Why we need to set boundaries on our generosity. *Greater Good.* https://greatergood.berkeley.edu/article/item/why_we_need_to_set_boundaries_on_our_generosity

26. Aknin, L. B., Sandstrom, G. M., Dunn, E. W., & Norton, M. I. (2011). It's the recipient that counts: Spending money on strong social ties leads to greater happiness than spending on weak social ties. *PLoS ONE, 6*(2), e17018. https://doi.org/10.1371/journal.pone.0017018

27. Hopper, E. (2018, September 7). What type of kindness will make you happiest? *Greater Good.* https://greatergood.berkeley.edu/article/item/what_types_of_kindness_will_make_you_happiest

28. Choi, J. N. (2009). Collective dynamics of citizenship behaviour: What group characteristics promote group-level helping? *Journal of Management Studies, 46*(8), 1396–1420. https://doi.org/10.1111/j.1467-6486.2009.00851.x

29. Levine, M., Prosser, A., Evans, D., & Reicher, S. (2005). Identity and emergency intervention: How social group membership and inclusiveness of group boundaries shape helping behavior. *Personality and Social Psychology Bulletin, 31*(4), 443–453. https://doi.org/10.1177/0146167204271651

30. Aknin, L. B., Dunn, E. W., Whillans, A. V., Grant, A. M., & Norton, M. I. (2013). Making a difference matters: Impact unlocks the emotional benefits of prosocial spending. *Journal of Economic Behavior & Organization, 88,* 90–95. https://doi.org/10.1016/j.jebo.2013.01.008

31. Tiayon, S. B. (2020, March 2). Does your culture affect your motivation to be kind? *Greater Good.* https://greatergood.berkeley.edu/article/item/does_your_culture_affect_your_motivation_to_be_kind

CHAPTER 3

1. Snarey, J. (1991). Faith development, moral development, and nontheistic Judaism: A construct validity study. In W. M. Kurtines & J. L. Gewirtz (Eds.), *Handbook of moral behavior and development* (pp. 279–305). Psychology Press.

2. De Waal, F. B. M., & Preston, S. D. (2017). Mammalian empathy: Behavioural manifestations and neural basis. *Nature Reviews Neuroscience, 18*(8), 498–509. https://doi.org/10.1038/nrn.2017.72

3. Sahu, S. (2023). Experiencing others: The science of empathy. In S. Chetri, T. Dutta, M. K. Mandal, & P. Patnaik (Eds.), *Understanding happiness* (pp. 249–264). Springer. https://doi.org/10.1007/978-981-99-3493-5_11

4. Healey, M. L., & Grossman, M. (2018). Cognitive and affective perspective-taking: Evidence for shared and dissociable anatomical substrates. *Frontiers in Neurology, 9.* https://doi.org/10.3389/fneur.2018.00491

5. Shamay-Tsoory, S. (2015). The neuropsychology of empathy: Evidence from lesion studies. *Revue de Neuropsychologie, Neurosciences Cognitives et Cliniques, 7*(4), 237–243.

6. Suttie, J. (2019, February 1). Why the world needs an empathy revolution. *Greater Good.* https://greatergood.berkeley.edu/article/item/why_the_world_needs_an_empathy_revolution

7. Roth-Hanania, R., Davidov, M., & Zahn-Waxler, C. (2011). Empathy development from 8 to 16 months: Early signs of concern for others. *Infant Behavior and Development*, *34*(3), 447–458. https://doi.org/10.1016/j.infbeh.2011.04.007
8. Frith, U., & Frith, C. D. (2003). Development and neurophysiology of mentalizing. *Philosophical Transactions of the Royal Society B Biological Sciences*, *358*(1431), 459–473. https://doi.org/10.1098/rstb.2002.1218
9. Svetlova, M., Nichols, S. R., & Brownell, C. A. (2010). Toddlers' prosocial behavior: From instrumental to empathic to altruistic helping. *Child Development*, *81*(6), 1814–1827. https://doi.org/10.1111/j.1467-8624.2010.01512.x
10. Batson, C. D. (2011). *Altruism in humans*. Oxford University Press. https://doi.org/10.1093/acprof:oso/9780195341065.001.0001
11. Zaki, J. (2019). Empathy is a moral force. In K. Gray & J. Graham (Eds.), *Atlas of moral psychology* (pp. 49–58). Guilford Press.
12. Allen, S., & Suttie, J. (2015, December 21). How our brains make us generous. *Greater Good*. https://greatergood.berkeley.edu/article/item/how_our_brains_make_us_generous
13. Eisenberg, N., & Miller, P. A. (1987). The relation of empathy to prosocial and related behaviors. *Psychological Bulletin*, *101*(1), 91–119. https://doi.org/10.1037/0033-2909.101.1.91
14. Choi, D., Minote, N., Sekiya, T., & Watanuki, S. (2016). Relationships between trait empathy and psychological well-being in Japanese university students. *Psychology*, *07*(09), 1240–1247. https://doi.org/10.4236/psych.2016.79126
15. Ferguson, A. M., Cameron, C. D., & Inzlicht, M. (2021). When does empathy feel good? *Current Opinion in Behavioral Sciences*, *39*, 125–129. https://doi.org/10.1016/j.cobeha.2021.03.011
16. Morelli, S. A., Ong, D. C., Makati, R., Jackson, M. O., & Zaki, J. (2017). Empathy and well-being correlate with centrality in different social networks. *Proceedings of the National Academy of Sciences*, *114*(37), 9843–9847. https://doi.org/10.1073/pnas.1702155114
17. Morelli, S. A., Lee, I. A., Arnn, M. E., & Zaki, J. (2015). Emotional and instrumental support provision interact to predict well-being. *Emotion*, *15*(4), 484–493. https://doi.org/10.1037/emo0000084
18. Cohen, S., Schulz, M. S., Weiss, E., & Waldinger, R. J. (2012). Eye of the beholder: The individual and dyadic contributions of empathic accuracy and perceived empathic effort to relationship satisfaction. *Journal of Family Psychology*, *26*(2), 236–245. https://doi.org/10.1037/a0027488
19. Scott, B. A., Colquitt, J. A., Paddock, E. L., & Judge, T. A. (2010). A daily investigation of the role of manager empathy on employee well-being. *Organizational Behavior and Human Decision Processes*, *113*(2), 127–140. https://doi.org/10.1016/j.obhdp.2010.08.001
20. Riess, H., Kelley, J. M., Bailey, R. W., Dunn, E. J., & Phillips, M. (2012). Empathy training for resident physicians: A randomized controlled trial of a neuroscience-informed curriculum. *Journal of General Internal Medicine*, *27*(10), 1280–1286. https://doi.org/10.1007/s11606-012-2063-z

21. Stewart, M. A. (1995). Effective physician-patient communication and health outcomes: A review. *CMAJ, 152*(9): 1423–1433.
22. Yue, Z., Qin, Y., Li, Y., Wang, J., Nicholas, S., Maitland, E., & Liu, C. (2022). Empathy and burnout in medical staff: Mediating role of job satisfaction and job commitment. *BMC Public Health, 22*(1). https://doi.org/10.1186/s12889-022-13405-4
23. Dixon, A. (2011, July 21). Can empathy reduce racism? *Greater Good.* https://greatergood.berkeley.edu/article/item/empathy_reduces_racism/
24. Pettigrew, T. F., & Tropp, L. R. (2008). How does intergroup contact reduce prejudice? Meta-analytic tests of three mediators. *European Journal of Social Psychology, 38*(6), 922–934. https://doi.org/10.1002/ejsp.504
25. Batson, C. D., Chang, J., Orr, R., & Rowland, J. (2002). Empathy, attitudes, and action: Can feeling for a member of a stigmatized group motivate one to help the group? *Personality and Social Psychology Bulletin, 28*(12), 1656–1666. https://doi.org/10.1177/014616702237647
26. Morelli, S. A., Lieberman, M. D., & Zaki, J. (2015). The emerging study of positive empathy. *Social and Personality Psychology Compass, 9*(2), 57–68. https://doi.org/10.1111/spc3.12157
27. Zaki, J. (2014). Empathy: A motivated account. *Psychological Bulletin, 140*(6), 1608–1647. https://doi.org/10.1037/a0037679
28. *Empathy quiz.* (2014, August). Greater Good. https://greatergood.berkeley.edu/quizzes/take_quiz/empathy
29. Weger, H., Castle Bell, G., Minei, E. M., & Robinson, M. C. (2014). The relative effectiveness of active listening in initial interactions. *International Journal of Listening, 28*(1), 13–31. https://doi.org/10.1080/10904018.2013.813234
30. Kuhn, R., Bradbury, T. N., Nussbeck, F. W., & Bodenmann, G. (2018). The power of listening: Lending an ear to the partner during dyadic coping conversations. *Journal of Family Psychology, 32*(6), 762–772. https://doi.org/10.1037/fam0000421
31. Suttie, J. (2021, August 31). How small moments of empathy affect your life. *Greater Good.* https://greatergood.berkeley.edu/article/item/how_small_moments_of_empathy_affect_your_life
32. Suttie, J. (2018, May 22). How putting yourself in someone else's shoes may backfire. *Greater Good.* https://greatergood.berkeley.edu/article/item/how_putting_yourself_in_someone_elses_shoes_may_backfire
33. Suttie, J. (2014, November 21). Why empathy matters. *Greater Good.* https://greatergood.berkeley.edu/article/item/why_empathy_matters
34. Suttie, J. (2022, August 30). Is your empathy biased? *Greater Good.* https://greatergood.berkeley.edu/article/item/is_your_empathy_biased
35. Svoboda, E. (2020, November 11). For a more empathic world, people have to choose empathy. *Greater Good.* https://greatergood.berkeley.edu/article/item/for_a_more_empathic_world_people_have_to_choose_empathy

36. Eva, A. L. (2017, May 4). How to stay empathic without suffering so much. *Greater Good*. https://greatergood.berkeley.edu/article/item/how_to_stay_empathic_without_suffering_so_much
37. Eva, A. L. (2017, May 4). How to stay empathic without suffering so much. *Greater Good*. https://greatergood.berkeley.edu/article/item/how_to_stay_empathic_without_suffering_so_much
38. Depow, G. J., Francis, Z., & Inzlicht, M. (2021). The experience of empathy in everyday life. *Psychological Science*, *32*(8), 1198–1213. https://doi.org/10.1177/0956797621995202
39. Azevedo, R. T., Macaluso, E., Avenanti, A., Santangelo, V., Cazzato, V., & Aglioti, S. M. (2012). Their pain is not our pain: Brain and autonomic correlates of empathic resonance with the pain of same and different race individuals. *Human Brain Mapping*, *34*(12), 3168–3181. https://doi.org/10.1002/hbm.22133
40. Saxton, K., Marsh, J., & Saslow, L. (2010, July 9). Do our brains think some people deserve to suffer? *Greater Good*. https://greatergood.berkeley.edu/article/research_digest/do_our_brains_think_some_people_deserve_to_suffer/
41. Preston, S. D., & De Waal, F. B. M. (2002). Empathy: Its ultimate and proximate bases. *Behavioral and Brain Sciences*, *25*(1), 1–20. https://doi.org/10.1017/s0140525x02000018
42. Van Bavel, J. J., Packer, D. J., & Cunningham, W. A. (2008). The neural substrates of in-group bias: A functional magnetic resonance imaging investigation. *Psychological Science*, *19*(11), 1131–1139. https://doi.org/10.1111/j.1467-9280.2008.02214.x
43. Leeuwen, E. van, & Mashuri, A. (2012). When common identities reduce between-group helping. *Social Psychological and Personality Science*, *3*(3), 259–265. https://doi.org/10.1177/1948550611417315
44. Newman, K. M., Lorenz, B., Klein, L., Bennett, L., Suttie, J., Smith, J. A., & Marsh, J. (2014, December 26). The top 10 insights from the "science of a meaningful life" in 2014. *Greater Good*. https://greatergood.berkeley.edu/article/item/the_top_ten_insights_from_the_science_of_a_meaningful_life_2014

CHAPTER 4

1. Seppälä, E. (2013, July 24). Compassionate mind, healthy body. *Greater Good*. https://greatergood.berkeley.edu/article/item/compassionate_mind_healthy_body
2. Goetz, J. L., Keltner, D., & Simon-Thomas, E. (2010). Compassion: An evolutionary analysis and empirical review. *Psychological Bulletin*, *136*(3), 351–374. https://doi.org/10.1037/a0018807
3. Keltner, D. (2012, July 31). The compassionate species. *Greater Good*. https://greatergood.berkeley.edu/article/item/the_compassionate_species
4. Gutkowska, J., Jankowski, M., Lambert, C., Mukaddam-Daher, S., Zingg, H. H., & McCann, S. M. (1997). Oxytocin releases atrial natriuretic peptide by combining with

oxytocin receptors in the heart. *Proceedings of the National Academy of Sciences, 94*(21), 11704–11709. https://doi.org/10.1073/pnas.94.21.11704

5. Love, T. M. (2014). Oxytocin, motivation and the role of dopamine. *Pharmacology Biochemistry and Behavior, 119*, 49–60. https://doi.org/10.1016/j.pbb.2013.06.011

6. Poehlmann-Tynan, J., Engbretson, A., Vigna, A. B., Weymouth, L. A., Burnson, C., Zahn-Waxler, C., Kapoor, A., Gerstein, E. D., Fanning, K. A., & Raison, C. L. (2019). Cognitively-Based Compassion Training for parents reduces cortisol in infants and young children. *Infant Mental Health Journal, 41*(1), 126–144. https://doi.org/10.1002/imhj.21831

7. Weng, H. Y., Fox, A. S., Shackman, A. J., Stodola, D. E., Caldwell, J. Z. K., Olson, M. C., Rogers, G. M., & Davidson, R. J. (2013). Compassion training alters altruism and neural responses to suffering. *Psychological Science, 24*(7), 1171–1180. https://doi.org/10.1177/0956797612469537

8. Goetz, J. L., Keltner, D., & Simon-Thomas, E. (2010). Compassion: An evolutionary analysis and empirical review. *Psychological Bulletin, 136*(3), 351–374. https://doi.org/10.1037/a0018807

9. Suttie, J. (2006, March 1). Compassion across cubicles. *Greater Good.* https://greatergood.berkeley.edu/article/item/compassion_across_cubicles

10. Klimecki, O. M., Leiberg, S., Lamm, C., & Singer, T. (2012). Functional neural plasticity and associated changes in positive affect after compassion training. *Cerebral Cortex, 23*(7), 1552–1561. https://doi.org/10.1093/cercor/bhs142

11. Brito-Pons, G., Campos, D., & Cebolla, A. (2018). Implicit or explicit compassion? Effects of Compassion Cultivation Training and comparison with Mindfulness-Based Stress Reduction. *Mindfulness, 9*(5), 1494–1508. https://doi.org/10.1007/s12671-018-0898-z

12. Lo, H. H. M., Ng, S. M., & Chan, C. L. W. (2014). Evaluating compassion–mindfulness therapy for recurrent anxiety and depression: A randomized control trial. *Research on Social Work Practice, 25*(6), 715–725. https://doi.org/10.1177/1049731514537686

13. Lang, A. J., Malaktaris, A. L., Casmar, P., Baca, S. A., Golshan, S., Harrison, T., & Negi, L. (2019). Compassion meditation for posttraumatic stress disorder in veterans: A randomized proof of concept study. *Journal of Traumatic Stress, 32*(2), 299–309. https://doi.org/10.1002/jts.22397

14. Lee, M. Y., Zaharlick, A., & Akers, D. (2015). Impact of meditation on mental health outcomes of female trauma survivors of interpersonal violence with co-occurring disorders: A randomized controlled trial. *Journal of Interpersonal Violence, 32*(14), 2139–2165. https://doi.org/10.1177/0886260515591277

15. Di Bello, M., Carnevali, L., Petrocchi, N., Thayer, J. F., Gilbert, P., & Ottaviani, C. (2020). The compassionate vagus: A meta-analysis on the connection between compassion and heart rate variability. *Neuroscience & Biobehavioral Reviews, 116*, 21–30. https://doi.org/10.1016/j.neubiorev.2020.06.016

16. Cosley, B. J., McCoy, S. K., Saslow, L. R., & Epel, E. S. (2010). Is compassion for others stress

buffering? Consequences of compassion and social support for physiological reactivity to stress. *Journal of Experimental Social Psychology, 46*(5), 816–823. https://doi.org/10.1016/j.jesp.2010.04.008

17. Ironson, G., Kremer, H., & Lucette, A. (2017). Compassionate love predicts long-term survival among people living with HIV followed for up to 17 years. *The Journal of Positive Psychology*, 1–10. https://doi.org/10.1080/17439760.2017.1350742

18. Pommier, E., Neff, K. D., & Tóth-Király I. (2019). The development and validation of the Compassion Scale. *Assessment*, 21–39.

19. Weng, H. Y., Fox, A. S., Shackman, A. J., Stodola, D. E., Caldwell, J. Z. K., Olson, M. C., Rogers, G. M., & Davidson, R. J. (2013). Compassion training alters altruism and neural responses to suffering. *Psychological Science, 24*(7), 1171–1180. http://dx.doi.org/10.1177/0956797612469537

20. Mak, W. W., Tong, A. C., Yip, S. Y., Lui, W. W., Chio, F. H., Chan, A. T., & Wong, C. C. (2018). Efficacy and moderation of mobile app-based programs for mindfulness-based training, self-compassion training, and cognitive behavioral psychoeducation on mental health: Randomized controlled noninferiority trial. *JMIR Mental Health, 5*(4), e60. https://doi.org/10.2196/mental.8597

21. Hwang, W. C., & Chan, C. P. (2019). Compassionate meditation to heal from race-related stress: A pilot study with Asian Americans. *American Journal of Orthopsychiatry, 89*(4), 482–492. http://doi.org/10.1037/ort0000372

22. Matos, M., Duarte, C., Duarte, J., Pinto-Gouveia, J., Petrocchi, N., Basran, J., & Gilbert, P. (2017). Psychological and physiological effects of compassionate mind training: A pilot randomised controlled study. *Mindfulness, 8*(6), 1699–1712. http://doi.org/10.1007/s12671-017-0745-7

23. Mikulincer, M., Shaver, P. R., Gillath, O., & Nitzberg, R. A. (2005). Attachment, caregiving, and altruism: Boosting attachment security increases compassion and helping. *Journal of Personality and Social Psychology, 89*(5), 817–839. https://doi.org/10.1037/0022-3514.89.5.817

24. Keltner, D. (2010, September 29). Hands on research: The science of touch. *Greater Good*. https://greatergood.berkeley.edu/article/item/hands_on_research/

25. Svoboda, E. (2021, May 3). What does "tough compassion" look like in real life? *Greater Good*. https://greatergood.berkeley.edu/article/item/what_does_tough_compassion_look_like_in_real_life

26. Eyal, N., & Worline, M. (2017, January 5). What does a compassionate workplace look like? *Greater Good*. https://greatergood.berkeley.edu/article/item/what_does_compassionate_workplace_look_like

27. Hanson, R. (2014, April 2). Just one thing: Recognize suffering in others. *Greater Good*. https://greatergood.berkeley.edu/article/item/just_one_thing_recognize_suffering_in_others

28. Jazaieri, H. (2018, April 24). Six habits of highly compassionate people. *Greater Good*. https://greatergood.berkeley.edu/article/item/six_habits_of_highly_compassionate_people
29. Cameron, C. D. (2013, January 16). How to increase your compassion bandwidth. *Greater Good*. https://greatergood.berkeley.edu/article/item/how_to_increase_your_compassion_bandwidth
30. Svoboda, E. (2022, April 7). How to deepen our compassion for refugees. *Greater Good*. https://greatergood.berkeley.edu/article/item/how_to_deepen_our_compassion_for_refugees
31. Svoboda, E. (2019, August 7). How to renew your compassion in the face of suffering. *Greater Good*. https://greatergood.berkeley.edu/article/item/how_to_renew_your_compassion_in_the_face_of_suffering
32. Simon-Thomas, E. R. (2019, November 18). Do your struggles expand your compassion for others? *Greater Good*. https://greatergood.berkeley.edu/article/item/do_your_struggles_expand_your_compassion_for_others
33. Svoboda, E. (2022, April 7). How to deepen our compassion for refugees. *Greater Good*. https://greatergood.berkeley.edu/article/item/how_to_deepen_our_compassion_for_refugees
34. Hanson, R. (2014b, September 26). Just one thing: Be at peace with the pain of others. *Greater Good*. https://greatergood.berkeley.edu/article/item/just_one_thing_be_at_peace_with_the_pain_of_others

CHAPTER 5

1. Cowen, A. S., & Keltner, D. (2021). Semantic space theory: A computational approach to emotion. *Trends in Cognitive Sciences, 25*(2), 124–136. https://doi.org/10.1016/j.tics.2020.11.004
2. Shiota, M. N., Neufeld, S. L., Yeung, W. H., Moser, S. E., & Perea, E. F. (2011). Feeling good: Autonomic nervous system responding in five positive emotions. *Emotion, 11*(6), 1368–1378. https://doi.org/10.1037/a0024278
3. Thomson, A. L., & Siegel, J. T. (2016). Elevation: A review of scholarship on a moral and other-praising emotion. *The Journal of Positive Psychology, 12*(6), 628–638. https://doi.org/10.1080/17439760.2016.1269184
4. Piff, P. K., Dietze, P., Feinberg, M., Stancato, D. M., & Keltner, D. (2015). Awe, the small self, and prosocial behavior. *Journal of Personality and Social Psychology, 108*(6), 883–899. https://doi.org/10.1037/pspi0000018
5. Stamkou, E., Brummelman, E., Dunham, R., Nikolic, M., & Keltner, D. (2023). Awe sparks prosociality in children. *Psychological Science, 34*(4), 455–467. https://doi.org/10.1177/09567976221150616
6. Piff, P. K., Dietze, P., Feinberg, M., Stancato, D. M., & Keltner, D. (2015). Awe, the small self, and prosocial behavior. *Journal of Personality and Social Psychology, 108*(6), 883–899. https://doi.org/10.1037/pspi0000018

7. Seo, M., Yang, S., & Laurent, S. M. (2023). No one is an island: Awe encourages global citizenship identification. *Emotion, 23*(3), 601–612. https://doi.org/10.1037/emo0001160
8. Bai, Y., Ocampo, J., Jin, G., Chen, S., Benet-Martinez, V., Monroy, M., Anderson, C., & Keltner, D. (2021). Awe, daily stress, and elevated life satisfaction. *Journal of Personality and Social Psychology, 120*(4), 837–860. https://doi.org/10.1037/pspa0000267
9. Rudd, M., Vohs, K. D., & Aaker, J. (2012). Awe expands people's perception of time, alters decision making, and enhances well-being. *Psychological Science, 23*(10), 1130–1136. https://doi.org/10.1177/0956797612438731
10. Nelson-Coffey, S. K., Ruberton, P. M., Chancellor, J., Cornick, J. E., Blascovich, J., & Lyubomirsky, S. (2019). The proximal experience of awe. *PLoS ONE, 14*(5), e0216780. https://doi.org/10.1371/journal.pone.0216780
11. Suttie, J. (2016, March 2). How nature can make you kinder, happier, and more creative. *Greater Good.* https://greatergood.berkeley.edu/article/item/how_nature_makes_you_kinder_happier_more_creative
12. Green, K., & Keltner, D. (2017, March 1). What happens when we reconnect with nature. *Greater Good.* https://greatergood.berkeley.edu/article/item/what_happens_when_we_reconnect_with_nature
13. Lopes, S., Lima, M., & Silva, K. (2020). Nature can get it out of your mind: The rumination reducing effects of contact with nature and the mediating role of awe and mood. *Journal of Environmental Psychology, 71*, 101489. https://doi.org/10.1016/j.jenvp.2020.101489
14. Anderson, C. L., Monroy, M., & Keltner, D. (2018). Awe in nature heals: Evidence from military veterans, at-risk youth, and college students. *Emotion, 18*(8), 1195–1202. https://doi.org/10.1037/emo0000442
15. Monroy, M., & Keltner, D. (2022). Awe as a pathway to mental and physical health. *Perspectives on Psychological Science, 18*(2), 309–320. https://doi.org/10.1177/17456916221094856
16. Monroy, M., Uğurlu, Ö., Zerwas, F., Corona, R., Keltner, D., Eagle, J., & Amster, M. (2023). The influences of daily experiences of awe on stress, somatic health, and well-being: A longitudinal study during COVID-19. *Scientific Reports, 13*(1). https://doi.org/10.1038/s41598-023-35200-w
17. Stellar, J. E., John-Henderson, N., Anderson, C. L., Gordon, A. M., McNeil, G. D., & Keltner, D. (2015). Positive affect and markers of inflammation: Discrete positive emotions predict lower levels of inflammatory cytokines. *Emotion, 15*(2), 129–133. https://doi.org/10.1037/emo0000033
18. Guan, F., Zhao, S., Chen, S., Lu, S., Chen, J., & Xiang, Y. (2019). The neural correlate difference between positive and negative awe. *Frontiers in Human Neuroscience, 13*. https://doi.org/10.3389/fnhum.2019.00206
19. Gordon, A. M., Stellar, J. E., Anderson, C. L., McNeil, G. D., Loew, D., & Keltner, D. (2017).

The dark side of the sublime: Distinguishing a threat-based variant of awe. *Journal of Personality and Social Psychology, 113*(2), 310–328. https://doi.org/10.1037/pspp0000120

20. Gordon, A. M., Stellar, J. E., Anderson, C. L., McNeil, G. D., Loew, D., & Keltner, D. (2017). The dark side of the sublime: Distinguishing a threat-based variant of awe. *Journal of Personality and Social Psychology, 113*(2), 310–328. https://doi.org/10.1037/pspp0000120
21. *Awe quiz*. (2016, May). Greater Good. https://greatergood.berkeley.edu/quizzes/take_quiz/awe
22. Sturm, V. E., Datta, S., Roy, A. R. K., Sible, I. J., Kosik, E. L., Veziris, C. R., Chow, T. E., Morris, N. A., Neuhaus, J., Kramer, J. H., Miller, B. L., Holley, S. R., & Keltner, D. (2022). Big smile, small self: Awe walks promote prosocial positive emotions in older adults. *Emotion, 22*(5), 1044–1058. https://doi.org/10.1037/emo0000876
23. Levasseur, A. (2023, September 8). How awe walks helped my students slow down. *Greater Good*. https://greatergood.berkeley.edu/article/item/how_awe_walks_helped_my_students_slow_down
24. Passmore, H., & Holder, M. D. (2016). Noticing nature: Individual and social benefits of a two-week intervention. *The Journal of Positive Psychology, 12*(6), 537–546. https://doi.org/10.1080/17439760.2016.1221126
25. Gordon, A. M., Stellar, J. E., Anderson, C. L., McNeil, G. D., Loew, D., & Keltner, D. (2017). The dark side of the sublime: Distinguishing a threat-based variant of awe. *Journal of Personality and Social Psychology, 113*(2), 310–328. https://doi.org/10.1037/pspp0000120
26. Keltner, D. (2020). *Awe: The new science of everyday wonder and how it can transform your life*. Penguin Press.
27. Keltner, D. (2023, January 24). What's the most common source of awe? *Greater Good*. https://greatergood.berkeley.edu/article/item/whats_the_most_common_source_of_awe
28. Stellar, J. E., Bai, Y., Anderson, C. L., Gordon, A., McNeil, G. D., Peng, K., & Keltner, D. (2024). Culture and awe: Understanding awe as a mixed emotion. *Affective Science, 5*(2), 160–170. https://doi.org/10.1007/s42761-024-00243-3
29. Stellar, J. E., Bai, Y., Anderson, C. L., Gordon, A., McNeil, G. D., Peng, K., & Keltner, D. (2024). Culture and awe: Understanding awe as a mixed emotion. *Affective Science, 5*(2), 160–170. https://doi.org/10.1007/s42761-024-00243-3
30. Bai, Y., Maruskin, L. A., Chen, S., Gordon, A. M., Stellar, J. E., McNeil, G. D., Peng, K., & Keltner, D. (2017). Awe, the diminished self, and collective engagement: Universals and cultural variations in the small self. *Journal of Personality and Social Psychology, 113*(2), 185–209. https://doi.org/10.1037/pspa0000087
31. Amster, M., & Eagle, J. (2020, April 15). Stuck at home? How to find awe and beauty indoors. *Greater Good*. https://greatergood.berkeley.edu/article/item/stuck_at_home_how_to_find_awe_beauty_indoors
32. Pattabhiraman, T. (2021, March 2). Six ways to incorporate awe into your daily life. *Greater*

Good. https://greatergood.berkeley.edu/article/item/six_ways_to_incorporate_awe_into_your_daily_life

33. BBC Earth. (2015, January 12). *Planet earth II* [Video]. YouTube. https://www.youtube.com/playlist?list=PL50KW6aT4UgzrIEk3rQjHCcHLayN1AbES

34. Amster, M., & Eagle, J. (2020, April 15). Stuck at home? How to find awe and beauty indoors. *Greater Good.* https://greatergood.berkeley.edu/article/item/stuck_at_home_how_to_find_awe_beauty_indoors

CHAPTER 6

1. Kabat-Zinn, J., Lipworth, L., & Burney, R. (1985). The clinical use of mindfulness meditation for the self-regulation of chronic pain. *Journal of Behavioral Medicine, 8*(2), 163–190. https://doi.org/10.1007/bf00845519

2. Borchardt, A. R., & Zoccola, P. M. (2018). Recovery from stress: An experimental examination of focused attention meditation in novices. *Journal of Behavioral Medicine, 41*(6), 836–849. https://doi.org/10.1007/s10865-018-9932-9

3. Ireland, M. J., Clough, B., Gill, K., Langan, F., O'Connor, A., & Spencer, L. (2017). A randomized controlled trial of mindfulness to reduce stress and burnout among intern medical practitioners. *Medical Teacher, 39*(4), 409–414. https://doi.org/10.1080/0142159x.2017.1294749

4. Liu, Z., Chen, Q. L., & Sun, Y. (2017). Mindfulness training for psychological stress in family caregivers of persons with dementia: A systematic review and meta-analysis of randomized controlled trials. *Clinical Interventions in Aging, 12,* 1521–1529. https://doi.org/10.2147/cia.s146213

5. Akman, Ö, & Yıldırım, D. (2023). The effect of mindfulness breathing-exercise on stress and depression symptoms in patients with chronic diseases. *Journal of Academic Research in Nursing, 9*(3), 197–204. https://doi.org/10.55646/jaren.2023.27576

6. Suttie, J. (2019, October 28). The mindfulness skill that is crucial for stress. *Greater Good.* https://greatergood.berkeley.edu/article/item/the_mindfulness_skill_that_is_crucial_for_stress

7. Burnett, D., Phillips, G., & Tashani, O. A. (2017). The effect of brief mindfulness meditation on cold-pressor induced pain responses in healthy adults. *Pain Studies and Treatment, 5*(2), 11–19. https://doi.org/10.4236/pst.2017.52002

8. Suttie, J. (2018, February 6). Could mindfulness help you control your anger? *Greater Good.* https://greatergood.berkeley.edu/article/item/could_mindfulness_help_you_control_your_anger

9. Roemer, L., Williston, S. K., & Rollins, L. G. (2015). Mindfulness and emotion regulation. *Current Opinion in Psychology, 3,* 52–57. https://doi.org/10.1016/j.copsyc.2015.02.006

10. Suttie, J. (2018, October 24). Five ways mindfulness meditation is good for your health.

Greater Good. https://greatergood.berkeley.edu/article/item/five_ways_mindfulness_meditation_is_good_for_your_health

11. Sünbül, Z. A., & Güneri, O. Y. (2019). The relationship between mindfulness and resilience: The mediating role of self compassion and emotion regulation in a sample of underprivileged Turkish adolescents. *Personality and Individual Differences*, *139*, 337–342. https://doi.org/10.1016/j.paid.2018.12.009

12. Davidson, R. J., Kabat-Zinn, J., Schumacher, J., Rosenkranz, M., Muller, D., Santorelli, S. F., Urbanowski, F., Harrington, A., Bonus, K., & Sheridan, J. F. (2003). Alterations in brain and immune function produced by mindfulness meditation. *Psychosomatic Medicine*, *65*(4), 564–570. https://doi.org/10.1097/01.psy.0000077505.67574.e3

13. Hülsheger, U. R., Feinholdt, A., & Nübold, A. (2015). A low-dose mindfulness intervention and recovery from work: Effects on psychological detachment, sleep quality, and sleep duration. *Journal of Occupational and Organizational Psychology*, *88*(3), 464–489. https://doi.org/10.1111/joop.12115

14. Suttie, J. (2023, December 4). Five ways mindfulness helps you age better. *Greater Good*. https://greatergood.berkeley.edu/article/item/five_ways_mindfulness_helps_you_age_better

15. Yip, D. (2017, May 18). How to tackle your cravings with mindfulness. *Greater Good*. https://greatergood.berkeley.edu/article/item/how_to_tackle_your_cravings_with_mindfulness

16. Shuai, R., Bakou, A. E., Hardy, L., & Hogarth, L. (2020). Ultra-brief breath counting (mindfulness) training promotes recovery from stress-induced alcohol-seeking in student drinkers. *Addictive Behaviors*, *102*, 106141. https://doi.org/10.1016/j.addbeh.2019.106141

17. Liu, F., Zhang, Z., Liu, S., & Feng, Z. (2022). Effectiveness of brief mindfulness intervention for college students' problematic smartphone use: The mediating role of self-control. *PLoS ONE*, *17*(12), e0279621. https://doi.org/10.1371/journal.pone.0279621

18. Kok, B. E., & Singer, T. (2016). Phenomenological fingerprints of four meditations: Differential state changes in affect, mind-wandering, meta-cognition, and interoception before and after daily practice across 9 months of training. *Mindfulness*, *8*(1), 218–231. https://doi.org/10.1007/s12671-016-0594-9

19. Miller, J. J., Fletcher, K., & Kabat-Zinn, J. (1995). Three-year follow-up and clinical implications of a mindfulness meditation-based stress reduction intervention in the treatment of anxiety disorders. *General Hospital Psychiatry*, *17*(3), 192–200. https://doi.org/10.1016/0163-8343(95)00025-m

20. Yip, D. (2020, January 10). Can mindfulness help when you're depressed? *Greater Good*. https://greatergood.berkeley.edu/article/item/can_mindfulness_help_when_youre_depressed

21. Segal, Z. V., Bieling, P., Young, T., MacQueen, G., Cooke, R., Martin, L., Bloch, R., &

Levitan, R. D. (2010). Antidepressant monotherapy vs sequential pharmacotherapy and mindfulness-based cognitive therapy, or placebo, for relapse prophylaxis in recurrent depression. *Archives of General Psychiatry, 67*(12), 1256. https://doi.org/10.1001/archgenpsychiatry.2010.168

22. Moore, A., Gruber, T., Derose, J., & Malinowski, P. (2012). Regular, brief mindfulness meditation practice improves electrophysiological markers of attentional control. *Frontiers in Human Neuroscience, 6.* https://doi.org/10.3389/fnhum.2012.00018

23. Levy, D. M., Wobbrock, J., Kaszniak, A. W., & Ostergren, M. (2012). The effects of mindfulness meditation training on multitasking in a high-stress information environment. *Proceedings of Graphics Interface 2012*, 45–52. https://graphicsinterface.org/proceedings/gi2012/gi2012-6/

24. Suttie, J. (2007, June 1). Mindful kids, peaceful schools. *Greater Good.* https://greatergood.berkeley.edu/article/item/mindful_kids_peaceful_schools

25. Roeser, R. W., Schonert-Reichl, K. A., Jha, A., Cullen, M., Wallace, L., Wilensky, R., Oberle, E., Thomson, K., Taylor, C., & Harrison, J. (2013). Mindfulness training and reductions in teacher stress and burnout: Results from two randomized, waitlist-control field trials. *Journal of Educational Psychology, 105*(3), 787–804. https://doi.org/10.1037/a0032093

26. Kerr, C. E., Jones, S. R., Wan, Q., Pritchett, D. L., Wasserman, R. H., Wexler, A., Villanueva, J. J., Shaw, J. R., Lazar, S. W., Kaptchuk, T. J., Littenberg, R., Hämäläinen, M. S., & Moore, C. I. (2011). Effects of mindfulness meditation training on anticipatory alpha modulation in primary somatosensory cortex. *Brain Research Bulletin, 85*(3–4), 96–103. https://doi.org/10.1016/j.brainresbull.2011.03.026

27. Henriksen, D., Gruber, N., & Woo, L. J. (2023, April 24). How mindfulness can help create calmer classrooms. *Greater Good.* https://greatergood.berkeley.edu/article/item/how_mindfulness_can_help_create_calmer_classrooms

28. Smith, J. A. (2014, November 17). Three benefits to mindfulness at work. *Greater Good.* https://greatergood.berkeley.edu/article/item/three_benefits_to_mindfulness_at_work

29. Shonin, E., Van Gordon, W., Slade, K., & Griffiths, M. D. (2013). Mindfulness and other Buddhist-derived interventions in correctional settings: A systematic review. *Aggression and Violent Behavior, 18*(3), 365–372. https://doi.org/10.1016/j.avb.2013.01.002

30. Hepner, K. A., Bloom, E. L., Newberry, S., Sousa, J. L., Osilla, K. C., Booth, M., Bialas, A., & Rutter, C. M. (2022). The impact of mindfulness meditation programs on performance-related outcomes: Implications for the U.S. army. *Rand Health Quarterly, 10*(1), 9.

31. Carson, J. W., Carson, K. M., Gil, K. M., & Baucom, D. H. (2004). Mindfulness-based relationship enhancement. *Behavior Therapy, 35*(3), 471–494. https://doi.org/10.1016/s0005-7894(04)80028-5

32. Dai, X., Du, N., Shi, S., & Lu, S. (2022). Effects of mindfulness-based interventions on peer relationships of children and adolescents: A systematic review and meta-analysis. *Mindfulness, 13*(11), 2653–2675. https://doi.org/10.1007/s12671-022-01966-9

33. Rizvi, S., Struthers, C. W., Shoikhedbrod, A., & Guilfoyle, J. R. (2022). Take a moment to apologize: How and why mindfulness affects apologies. *Journal of Experimental Psychology Applied*, 28(3), 661–675. https://doi.org/10.1037/xap0000387
34. Suttie, J. (2017, May 17). Three ways mindfulness can make you less biased. *Greater Good*. https://greatergood.berkeley.edu/article/item/three_ways_mindfulness_can_make_you_less_biased
35. Don, B. P. (2019). Mindfulness predicts growth belief and positive outcomes in social relationships. *Self and Identity*, 19(3), 272–292. https://doi.org/10.1080/15298868.2019.1571526
36. Hanley, A. W., & Garland, E. L. (2017). Clarity of mind: Structural equation modeling of associations between dispositional mindfulness, self-concept clarity and psychological well-being. *Personality and Individual Differences*, 106, 334–339. https://doi.org/10.1016/j.paid.2016.10.028
37. Christie, A. M., Atkins, P. W. B., & Donald, J. N. (2016). The meaning and doing of mindfulness: The role of values in the link between mindfulness and well-being. *Mindfulness*, 8(2), 368–378. https://doi.org/10.1007/s12671-016-0606-9
38. Marsh, J. (2013, May 23). How to train the compassionate brain. *Greater Good*. https://greatergood.berkeley.edu/article/item/how_to_train_the_compassionate_brain
39. Condon, P., Desbordes, G., Miller, W. B., & DeSteno, D. (2013). Meditation increases compassionate responses to suffering. *Psychological Science*, 24(10), 2125–2127. https://doi.org/10.1177/0956797613485603
40. *Mindfulness quiz*. (2011, September). Greater Good. https://greatergood.berkeley.edu/quizzes/take_quiz/mindfulness
41. Newman, K. M. (2016, October 11). How to choose a type of mindfulness meditation. *Greater Good*. https://greatergood.berkeley.edu/article/item/how_to_choose_a_type_of_mindfulness_meditation
42. Tsang, S. C., Mok, E. S., Lam, S. C., & Lee, J. K. (2012). The benefit of mindfulness-based stress reduction to patients with terminal cancer. *Journal of Clinical Nursing*, 21(17–18), 2690–2696. https://doi.org/10.1111/j.1365-2702.2012.04111.x
43. *UCLA mindful*. (n.d.). UCLA Health. Retrieved August 14, 2024, from http://marc.ucla.edu/
44. Newman, K. M. (2016, October 11). How to choose a type of mindfulness meditation. *Greater Good*.
45. Jazaieri, H. (2014, April 21). Which kind of mindfulness meditation is right for you? *Greater Good*. https://greatergood.berkeley.edu/article/item/which_kind_of_mindfulness_meditation_is_right_for_you
46. Simon-Thomas, E. R. (2022, September 14). Does mindfulness get in the way of making amends? *Greater Good*. https://greatergood.berkeley.edu/article/item/does_mindfulness_get_in_the_way_of_making_amends
47. Singer, T. (2018, July 2). What type of meditation is best for you? *Greater Good*. https://greatergood.berkeley.edu/article/item/what_type_of_meditation_is_best_for_you

48. Hougaard, R., & Carter, J. (2016, April 11). How to practice mindfulness throughout your work day. *Greater Good.* https://greatergood.berkeley.edu/article/item/how_to_practice_mindfulness_throughout_your_work_day
49. Hunt, C. (2022, March 22). Four tips for sticking to a meditation practice. *Greater Good.* https://greatergood.berkeley.edu/article/item/four_tips_for_sticking_to_a_meditation_practice
50. Kabat-Zinn, J. (2010, May). *The stars of our own movie* [Video]. Greater Good. https://greatergood.berkeley.edu/video/item/the_stars_of_our_own_movie
51. Weiss, L. (2016, January 21). Can we be mindful at work without meditating? *Greater Good.* https://greatergood.berkeley.edu/article/item/can_we_be_mindful_at_work_without_meditating
52. Hanley, A. W., Warner, A. R., Dehili, V. M., Canto, A. I., & Garland, E. L. (2014). Washing dishes to wash the dishes: Brief instruction in an informal mindfulness practice. *Mindfulness, 6*(5), 1095–1103. https://doi.org/10.1007/s12671-014-0360-9

CHAPTER 7

1. Watkins, P. C., Woodward, K., Stone, T., & Kolts, R. L. (2003). Gratitude and happiness: Development of a measure of gratitude, and relationships with subjective well-being. *Social Behavior and Personality an International Journal, 31*(5), 431–451. https://doi.org/10.2224/sbp.2003.31.5.431
2. Wang, L., Gonzalez, P. D., Lau, P. L., Vaughan, E. L., & Costa, M. F. (2023). "Dando gracias": Gratitude, social connectedness, and subjective happiness among bilingual Latinx college students. *Journal of Latinx Psychology, 11*(3), 203–219. https://doi.org/10.1037/lat0000227
3. Emmons, R. A., & McCullough, M. E. (2003). Counting blessings versus burdens: An experimental investigation of gratitude and subjective well-being in daily life. *Journal of Personality and Social Psychology, 84*(2), 377–389. https://doi.org/10.1037/0022-3514.84.2.377
4. Liao, K. Y., & Weng, C. (2018). Gratefulness and subjective well-being: Social connectedness and presence of meaning as mediators. *Journal of Counseling Psychology, 65*(3), 383–393. https://doi.org/10.1037/cou0000271
5. Elfers, J., Hlava, P., Sharpe, F., Arreguin, S., & McGregor, D. C. (2023). Resilience and loss: The correlation of grief and gratitude. *International Journal of Applied Positive Psychology, 9*(1), 327–345. https://doi.org/10.1007/s41042-023-00126-1
6. Algoe, S. B., & Stanton, A. L. (2012). Gratitude when it is needed most: Social functions of gratitude in women with metastatic breast cancer. *Emotion, 12*(1), 163–168. https://doi.org/10.1037/a0024024
7. Crouch, T. A., Verdi, E. K., & Erickson, T. M. (2020). Gratitude is positively associated

with quality of life in multiple sclerosis. *Rehabilitation Psychology, 65*(3), 231–238. https://doi.org/10.1037/rep0000319

8. Smith, J. A. (2014, November 26). Can giving thanks help us heal from trauma? *Greater Good.* https://greatergood.berkeley.edu/article/item/can_giving_thanks_help_heal_from_trauma

9. Kumar, S. A., Edwards, M. E., Grandgenett, H. M., Scherer, L. L., DiLillo, D., & Jaffe, A. E. (2022). Does gratitude promote resilience during a pandemic? An examination of mental health and positivity at the onset of COVID-19. *Journal of Happiness Studies, 23*(7), 3463–3483. https://doi.org/10.1007/s10902-022-00554-x

10. Kurian, R. M., & Thomas, S. (2023). Gratitude as a path to human prosperity during adverse circumstances: A narrative review. *British Journal of Guidance and Counselling, 51*(5), 739–752. https://doi.org/10.1080/03069885.2022.2154314

11. Emmons, R. (2013, May 13). How gratitude can help you through hard times. *Greater Good.* https://greatergood.berkeley.edu/article/item/how_gratitude_can_help_you_through_hard_times

12. Redwine, L. S., Henry, B. L., Pung, M. A., Wilson, K., Chinh, K., Knight, B., Jain, S., Rutledge, T., Greenberg, B., Maisel, A., & Mills, P. J. (2016). Pilot randomized study of a gratitude journaling intervention on heart rate variability and inflammatory biomarkers in patients with Stage B heart failure. *Psychosomatic Medicine, 78*(6), 667–676. https://doi.org/10.1097/psy.0000000000000316

13. Wood, A. M., Joseph, S., Lloyd, J., & Atkins, S. (2009). Gratitude influences sleep through the mechanism of pre-sleep cognitions. *Journal of Psychosomatic Research, 66*(1), 43–48. https://doi.org/10.1016/j.jpsychores.2008.09.002

14. Newman, K. M. (2017, September 6). How gratitude can transform your workplace. *Greater Good.* https://greatergood.berkeley.edu/article/item/how_gratitude_can_transform_your_workplace

15. Kyeong, S., Kim, J., Kim, D. J., Kim, H. E., & Kim, J. (2017). Effects of gratitude meditation on neural network functional connectivity and brain-heart coupling. *Scientific Reports, 7*(1). https://doi.org/10.1038/s41598-017-05520-9

16. Gordon, A. M., Impett, E. A., Kogan, A., Oveis, C., & Keltner, D. (2012). To have and to hold: Gratitude promotes relationship maintenance in intimate bonds. *Journal of Personality and Social Psychology, 103*(2), 257–274. https://doi.org/10.1037/a0028723

17. Lambert, N. M., Clark, M. S., Durtschi, J., Fincham, F. D., & Graham, S. M. (2010). Benefits of expressing gratitude: Expressing gratitude to a partner changes one's view of the relationship. *Psychological Science, 21*(4), 574–580. https://doi.org/10.1177/0956797610364003

18. Nelson-Coffey, S. K., & Coffey, J. K. (2024). Gratitude improves parents' well-being and family functioning. *Emotion, 24*(2), 357–369. https://doi.org/10.1037/emo0001283

19. Vaish, A., & Savell, S. (2022). Young children value recipients who display gratitude. *Developmental Psychology*, *58*(4), 680–692. https://doi.org/10.1037/dev0001308
20. Bono, G., & Froh, J. (2012, November 19). How to foster gratitude in schools. *Greater Good*. https://greatergood.berkeley.edu/article/item/how_to_foster_gratitude_in_schools
21. Ma, M., Kibler, J. L., & Sly, K. (2013). Gratitude is associated with greater levels of protective factors and lower levels of risks in African American adolescents. *Journal of Adolescence*, *36*(5), 983–991. https://doi.org/10.1016/j.adolescence.2013.07.012
22. Chamizo-Nieto, M. T., Wallace, A., & Rey, L. (2023). Anti-cyberbullying interventions at school: Comparing the effectiveness of gratitude and psychoeducational programmes. *The Journal of Positive Psychology*, *19*(2), 291–300. https://doi.org/10.1080/17439760.2023.2170821
23. Ma, L. K., Tunney, R. J., & Ferguson, E. (2017). Does gratitude enhance prosociality?: A meta-analytic review. *Psychological Bulletin*, *143*(6), 601–635. https://doi.org/10.1037/bul0000103
24. Bartlett, M. Y., & DeSteno, D. (2006). Gratitude and prosocial behavior. *Psychological Science*, *17*(4), 319–325. https://doi.org/10.1111/j.1467-9280.2006.01705.x
25. Armenta, C. N., & Lyubomirsky, S. (2017, May 23). How gratitude motivates us to become better people. *Greater Good*. https://greatergood.berkeley.edu/article/item/how_gratitude_motivates_us_to_become_better_people
26. Suttie, J. (2019b, December 20). The ripple effects of a thank you. *Greater Good*. https://greatergood.berkeley.edu/article/item/the_ripple_effects_of_a_thank_you
27. *Gratitude quiz*. (2011, November). Greater Good. https://greatergood.berkeley.edu/quizzes/take_quiz/gratitude
28. Seligman, M. E. P., Steen, T. A., Park, N., & Peterson, C. (2005). Positive psychology progress: Empirical validation of interventions. *American Psychologist*, *60*(5), 410–421. https://doi.org/10.1037/0003-066x.60.5.410
29. Froh, J. J., Kashdan, T. B., Ozimkowski, K. M., & Miller, N. (2009). Who benefits the most from a gratitude intervention in children and adolescents? Examining positive affect as a moderator. *The Journal of Positive Psychology*, *4*(5), 408–422. https://doi.org/10.1080/17439760902992464
30. Layous, K., Lee, H., Choi, I., & Lyubomirsky, S. (2013). Culture matters when designing a successful happiness-increasing activity: A comparison of the United States and South Korea. *Journal of Cross-Cultural Psychology*, *44*(8), 1294–1303. https://doi.org/10.1177/0022022113487591
31. Titova, L., Wagstaff, A. E., & Parks, A. C. (2017). Disentangling the effects of gratitude and optimism: A cross-cultural investigation. *Journal of Cross-Cultural Psychology*, *48*(5), 754–770. https://doi.org/10.1177/0022022117699278
32. Shin, L. J., Armenta, C. N., Kamble, S. V., Chang, S., Wu, H., & Lyubomirsky, S. (2020). Gratitude in collectivist and individualist cultures. *The Journal of Positive Psychology*, *15*(5), 598–604. https://doi.org/10.1080/17439760.2020.1789699

33. Titova, L., Wagstaff, A. E., & Parks, A. C. (2017). Disentangling the effects of gratitude and optimism: A cross-cultural investigation. *Journal of Cross-Cultural Psychology, 48*(5), 754–770. https://doi.org/10.1177/0022022117699278
34. Shin, L. J., Armenta, C. N., Kamble, S. V., Chang, S., Wu, H., & Lyubomirsky, S. (2020). Gratitude in collectivist and individualist cultures. *The Journal of Positive Psychology, 15*(5), 598–604. https://doi.org/10.1080/17439760.2020.1789699
35. Naito, T., & Sakata, Y. (2010). Gratitude, indebtedness, and regret on receiving a friend's favor in Japan. *Psychologia, 53*(3), 179–194. https://doi.org/10.2117/psysoc.2010.179
36. Smith, J. A. (2013, November 20). Six habits of highly grateful people. *Greater Good.* https://greatergood.berkeley.edu/article/item/six_habits_of_highly_grateful_people
37. Hanson, R. (2009, November 1). Taking in the good. *Greater Good.* https://greatergood.berkeley.edu/article/item/taking_in_the_good
38. Springer, A. (2018, January 22). Five ways to make the most of your gratitude. *Greater Good.* https://greatergood.berkeley.edu/article/item/five_ways_to_make_the_most_of_your_gratitude
39. Newman, Kira M. (2015, November 18). The trouble with Thanksgiving gratitude. *Greater Good.* https://greatergood.berkeley.edu/article/item/the_trouble_with_thanksgiving_gratitude
40. Emmons, R. (2010, November 17). 10 ways to become more grateful. *Greater Good.* https://greatergood.berkeley.edu/article/item/ten_ways_to_become_more_grateful1
41. Emmons, R. (2010, November). *Cultivating gratitude* [Video]. Greater Good. https://greatergood.berkeley.edu/video/item/cultivating_gratitude
42. Emmons, R. (2013b, May 13). How gratitude can help you through hard times. *Greater Good.* https://greatergood.berkeley.edu/article/item/how_gratitude_can_help_you_through_hard_times
43. Allen, S. (2018, August 15). Do men have a gratitude problem? *Greater Good.* https://greatergood.berkeley.edu/article/item/do_men_have_a_gratitude_problem

CHAPTER 8

1. Brooks, R. (2021, July 22). Who is René Brooks? *Black Girl, Lost Keys.* https://blackgirllostkeys.com/rene-brooks/
2. Neff, K. D., & Vonk, R. (2008). Self-compassion versus global self-esteem: Two different ways of relating to oneself. *Journal of Personality, 77*(1), 23–50. https://doi.org/10.1111/j.1467-6494.2008.00537.x
3. Neff, K. D., Kirkpatrick, K. L., & Rude, S. S. (2007). Self-compassion and adaptive psychological functioning. *Journal of Research in Personality, 41*(1), 139–154. https://doi.org/10.1016/j.jrp.2006.03.004
4. Arch, J. J., Brown, K. W., Dean, D. J., Landy, L. N., Brown, K. D., & Laudenslager, M. L. (2014). Self-compassion training modulates alpha-amylase, heart rate variability, and

subjective responses to social evaluative threat in women. *Psychoneuroendocrinology, 42*, 49–58. https://doi.org/10.1016/j.psyneuen.2013.12.018

5. Helminen, E. C., Ducar, D. M., Scheer, J. R., Parke, K. L., Morton, M. L., & Felver, J. C. (2023). Self-compassion, minority stress, and mental health in sexual and gender minority populations: A meta-analysis and systematic review. *Clinical Psychology Science and Practice, 30*(1), 26–39. https://doi.org/10.1037/cps0000104

6. Hiraoka, R., Meyer, E. C., Kimbrel, N. A., DeBeer, B. B., Gulliver, S. B., & Morissette, S. B. (2015). Self-compassion as a prospective predictor of PTSD symptom severity among trauma-exposed U.S. Iraq and Afghanistan war veterans. *Journal of Traumatic Stress, 28*(2), 127–133. https://doi.org/10.1002/jts.21995

7. Phelps, C. L., Paniagua, S. M., Willcockson, I. U., & Potter, J. S. (2018). The relationship between self-compassion and the risk for substance use disorder. *Drug and Alcohol Dependence, 183*, 78–81. https://doi.org/10.1016/j.drugalcdep.2017.10.026

8. Rodgers, R. F., Franko, D. L., Donovan, E., Cousineau, T., Yates, K., McGowan, K., Cook, E., & Lowy, A. S. (2017). Body image in emerging adults: The protective role of self-compassion. *Body Image, 22*, 148–155. https://doi.org/10.1016/j.bodyim.2017.07.003

9. Van Dam, N. T., Sheppard, S. C., Forsyth, J. P., & Earleywine, M. (2011). Self-compassion is a better predictor than mindfulness of symptom severity and quality of life in mixed anxiety and depression. *Journal of Anxiety Disorders, 25*(1), 123–130. https://doi.org/10.1016/j.janxdis.2010.08.011

10. Diedrich, A., Grant, M., Hofmann, S. G., Hiller, W., & Berking, M. (2014). Self-compassion as an emotion regulation strategy in major depressive disorder. *Behaviour Research and Therapy, 58*, 43–51. https://doi.org/10.1016/j.brat.2014.05.006

11. Sotiropoulou, K., Patitsa, C., Giannakouli, V., Galanakis, M., Koundourou, C., & Tsitsas, G. (2023). Self-compassion as a key factor of subjective happiness and psychological well-being among Greek adults during COVID-19 lockdowns. *International Journal of Environmental Research and Public Health, 20*(15), 6464. https://doi.org/10.3390/ijerph20156464

12. Lathren, C. R., Rao, S. S., Park, J., & Bluth, K. (2021). Self-compassion and current close interpersonal relationships: A scoping literature review. *Mindfulness, 12*(5), 1078–1093. https://doi.org/10.1007/s12671-020-01566-5

13. Yarnell, L. M., & Neff, K. D. (2013). Self-compassion, interpersonal conflict resolutions, and well-being. *Self and Identity, 12*(2), 146–159. https://doi.org/10.1080/15298868.2011.649545

14. Neff, K. D., & Beretvas, S. N. (2013). The role of self-compassion in romantic relationships. *Self and Identity, 12*(1), 78–98. https://doi.org/10.1080/15298868.2011.639548

15. Vu, H. A., & Rivera, L. M. (2022). Self-compassion and negative outgroup attitudes: The mediating role of compassion for others. *Self and Identity, 22*(3), 470–485. https://doi.org/10.1080/15298868.2022.2117241

16. Neff, K. (2015, September 30). The five myths of self-compassion. *Greater Good.* https://greatergood.berkeley.edu/article/item/the_five_myths_of_self_compassion
17. Breines, J. G., & Chen, S. (2012). Self-compassion increases self-improvement motivation. *Personality and Social Psychology Bulletin, 38*(9), 1133–1143. https://doi.org/10.1177/0146167212445599
18. Liao, K. Y., Stead, G. B., & Liao, C. (2021). A meta-analysis of the relation between self-compassion and self-efficacy. *Mindfulness, 12*(8), 1878–1891. https://doi.org/10.1007/s12671-021-01626-4
19. Long, P. (2018, January 3). Make self-compassion one of your New Year's resolutions. *Greater Good.* https://greatergood.berkeley.edu/article/item/make_self_compassion_one_of_your_new_years_resolutions
20. Zessin, U., Dickhäuser, O., & Garbade, S. (2015). The relationship between self-compassion and well-being: A meta-analysis. *Health and Well-Being, 7*(3), 340–364. https://iaap-journals.onlinelibrary.wiley.com/doi/10.1111/aphw.12051
21. *Self-compassion quiz.* (2021, June). Greater Good. https://greatergood.berkeley.edu/quizzes/take_quiz/self_compassion
22. Shapira, L. B., & Mongrain, M. (2010). The benefits of self-compassion and optimism exercises for individuals vulnerable to depression. *The Journal of Positive Psychology, 5*(5), 377–389. https://doi.org/10.1080/17439760.2010.516763
23. Breines, J., & Chen, S. (2013). Activating the inner caregiver: The role of support-giving schemas in increasing state self-compassion. *Journal of Experimental Social Psychology, 49,* 58–64. https://doi.org/10.1016/j.jesp.2012.07.015
24. Benner, C. (2022, October 26). Why is self-compassion so hard for some people? *Greater Good.* https://greatergood.berkeley.edu/article/item/why_is_self_compassion_so_hard_for_some_people
25. Desmond, T. (2016, January 27). Five ways to put self-compassion into therapy. *Greater Good.* https://greatergood.berkeley.edu/article/item/five_ways_to_put_self_compassion_into_therapy
26. Weiss, L. (2018, March 15). How to bring self-compassion to work with you. *Greater Good.* https://greatergood.berkeley.edu/article/item/how_to_bring_self_compassion_to_work_with_you
27. Newman, K. M. (2018, March 2). What self-compassion feels like in your body. *Greater Good.* https://greatergood.berkeley.edu/article/item/what_self_compassion_feels_like_in_your_body
28. Benner, C. (2022, October 26). Why is self-compassion so hard for some people? *Greater Good.* https://greatergood.berkeley.edu/article/item/why_is_self_compassion_so_hard_for_some_people
29. Benner, C. (2022, October 26). Why is self-compassion so hard for some people? *Greater*

Good. https://greatergood.berkeley.edu/article/item/why_is_self_compassion_so_hard_for_some_people

30. Center for Mindful Self-Compassion. (n.d.). *Self-compassion in daily life*. Chris Germer. Retrieved August 15, 2024, from https://chrisgermer.com/wp-content/uploads/2020/11/Self-Compassion-in-Daily-Life.pdf
31. Neff, K. (2018, October 17). Why women need fierce self-compassion. *Greater Good*. https://greatergood.berkeley.edu/article/item/why_women_need_fierce_self_compassion
32. *Fierce self-compassion break*. (2021, June). Greater Good in Action. https://ggia.berkeley.edu/practice/fierce_self_compassion_break
33. Ewert, C., Vater, A., & Schröder-Abé, M. (2021). Self-compassion and coping: A meta-analysis. *Mindfulness, 12*(5), 1063–1077. https://doi.org/10.1007/s12671-020-01563-8
34. Chan, K. K. S., Yung, C. S. W., & Nie, G. M. (2020). Self-compassion buffers the negative psychological impact of stigma stress on sexual minorities. *Mindfulness, 11*(10), 2338–2348. https://doi.org/10.1007/s12671-020-01451-1
35. Vigna, A. J., Poehlmann-Tynan, J., & Koenig, B. W. (2017). Does self-compassion facilitate resilience to stigma? A school-based study of sexual and gender minority youth. *Mindfulness, 9*(3), 914–924. https://doi.org/10.1007/s12671-017-0831-x

CHAPTER 9

1. Damasio, A. R. (2022, February 8). *Keynote address: "The science of emotion."* Library of Congress. Retrieved May 1, 2024, from https://www.loc.gov/loc/brain/emotion/Damasio.html
2. Karnaze, M. M., & Levine, L. J. (2017). Data versus Spock: Lay theories about whether emotion helps or hinders. *Cognition & Emotion, 32*(3), 549–565. https://doi.org/10.1080/02699931.2017.1326374
3. Ford, B. Q., Lam, P., John, O. P., & Mauss, I. B. (2018). The psychological health benefits of accepting negative emotions and thoughts: Laboratory, diary, and longitudinal evidence. *Journal of Personality and Social Psychology, 115*(6), 1075–1092. https://doi.org/10.1037/pspp0000157
4. Bailen, N., Thompson, R., & Hallenbeck, H. W. (2018, November 26). How to deal with feeling bad about your feelings. *Greater Good*. https://greatergood.berkeley.edu/article/item/how_to_deal_with_feeling_bad_about_your_feelings
5. Farb, N. A. S., Anderson, A. K., & Segal, Z. V. (2012). The mindful brain and emotion regulation in mood disorders. *The Canadian Journal of Psychiatry, 57*(2), 70–77. https://doi.org/10.1177/070674371205700203
6. Hofmann, S. G., Sawyer, A. T., Witt, A. A., & Oh, D. (2010). The effect of mindfulness-based therapy on anxiety and depression: A meta-analytic review. *Journal of Consulting and Clinical Psychology, 78*(2), 169–183. https://doi.org/10.1037/a0018555
7. Jamieson, J. P., Nock, M. K., & Mendes, W. B. (2012). Mind over matter: Reappraising

arousal improves cardiovascular and cognitive responses to stress. *Journal of Experimental Psychology General*, *141*(3), 417–422. https://doi.org/10.1037/a0025719

8. Suttie, J. (2023, February 15). Seven ways to have a healthier relationship with stress. *Greater Good.* https://greatergood.berkeley.edu/article/item/seven_ways_to_have_a_healthier_relationship_with_stress

9. Smith, E. N., Romero, C., Donovan, B., Herter, R., Paunesku, D., Cohen, G. L., Dweck, C. S., & Gross, J. J. (2018). Emotion theories and adolescent well-being: Results of an online intervention. *Emotion*, *18*(6), 781–788. https://doi.org/10.1037/emo0000379

10. Suttie, J. (2021, June 21). Does venting your feelings actually help? *Greater Good.* https://greatergood.berkeley.edu/article/item/does_venting_your_feelings_actually_help

11. Malinauskas, R., & Malinauskiene, V. (2020). The relationship between emotional intelligence and psychological well-being among male university students: The mediating role of perceived social support and perceived stress. *International Journal of Environmental Research and Public Health*, *17*(5), 1605. https://doi.org/10.3390/ijerph17051605

12. Schneider, T. R., Lyons, J. B., & Khazon, S. (2013). Emotional intelligence and resilience. *Personality and Individual Differences*, *55*(8), 909–914. https://doi.org/10.1016/j.paid.2013.07.460

13. Collado-Soler, R., Trigueros, R., Aguilar-Parra, J. M., & Navarro, N. (2023). Emotional intelligence and resilience outcomes in adolescent period, is knowledge really strength? *Psychology Research and Behavior Management*, *16*, 1365–1378. https://doi.org/10.2147/prbm.s383296

14. *Adaptive coping.* (n.d.). ScienceDirect. https://www.sciencedirect.com/topics/psychology/adaptive-coping

15. Kross, E., & Ayduk, O. (2017). Self-distancing: theory, research, and current directions. In J. M. Olson (Ed.), *Advances in experimental social psychology* (pp. 81–136). Academic Press. https://doi.org/10.1016/bs.aesp.2016.10.002

16. Stoeber, J., & Janssen, D. P. (2011). Perfectionism and coping with daily failures: Positive reframing helps achieve satisfaction at the end of the day. *Anxiety, Stress, & Coping*, *24*(5), 477–497. https://doi.org/10.1080/10615806.2011.562977

17. Robbins, M. L., Wright, R. C., López, A. M., & Weihs, K. (2019). Interpersonal positive reframing in the daily lives of couples coping with breast cancer. *Journal of Psychosocial Oncology*, *37*(2), 160–177. https://doi.org/10.1080/07347332.2018.1555198

18. Ozbay, F., Johnson, D. C., Dimoulas, E., Morgan, III, C. A., Charney, D., & Southwick, S. (2007). Social support and resilience to stress: From neurobiology to clinical practice. *Psychiatry (Edgmont)*, *4*(5), 35–40. https://pubmed.ncbi.nlm.nih.gov/20806028

19. Brackett, M. A., Rivers, S. E., Bertoli, M. C., & Salovey, P. (2016). Emotional intelligence. In L. F. Barrett, M. Lewis, & J. M. Haviland-Jones (Eds.), *Handbook of emotions* (pp. 513–531). Guilford Publications.

20. Höfmann, S. G., & Kashdan, T. B. (2009). The Affective Style Questionnaire: Development and psychometric properties. *Journal of Psychopathology and Behavioral Assessment, 32*(2), 255–263. https://doi.org/10.1007/s10862-009-9142-4
21. DiMenichi, B. C., Lempert, K. M., Bejjani, C., & Tricomi, E. (2018). Writing about past failures attenuates cortisol responses and sustained attention deficits following psychosocial stress. *Frontiers in Behavioral Neuroscience, 12*. https://doi.org/10.3389/fnbeh.2018.00045
22. Qian, J., Zhou, X., Sun, X., Wu, M., Sun, S., & Yu, X. (2020). Effects of expressive writing intervention for women's PTSD, depression, anxiety and stress related to pregnancy: A meta-analysis of randomized controlled trials. *Psychiatry Research, 288*, 112933. https://doi.org/10.1016/j.psychres.2020.112933
23. Zhou, C., Wu, Y., An, S., & Li, X. (2015). Effect of expressive writing intervention on health outcomes in breast cancer patients: A systematic review and meta-analysis of randomized controlled trials. *PLoS ONE, 10*(7), e0131802. https://doi.org/10.1371/journal.pone.0131802
24. Oh, P., & Kim, S. H. (2016). The effects of expressive writing interventions for patients with cancer: A meta-analysis. *Oncology Nursing Forum, 43*(4), 468–479. https://doi.org/10.1188/16.onf.468-479
25. Abu-Odah, H., Su, J. J., Wang, M., Sheffield, D., & Molassiotis, A. (2023). Systematic review and meta-analysis of the effectiveness of expressive writing disclosure on cancer and palliative care patients' health-related outcomes. *Supportive Care in Cancer, 32*(1). https://doi.org/10.1007/s00520-023-08255-8
26. Frisina, P. G., Borod, J. C., & Lepore, S. J. (2004). A meta-analysis of the effects of written emotional disclosure on the health outcomes of clinical populations. *The Journal of Nervous and Mental Disease, 192*(9), 629–634. https://doi.org/10.1097/01.nmd.0000138317.30764.63
27. Guo, L. (2022). The delayed, durable effect of expressive writing on depression, anxiety and stress: A meta-analytic review of studies with long-term follow-ups. *British Journal of Clinical Psychology, 62*(1), 272–297. https://doi.org/10.1111/bjc.12408
28. Reinhold, M., Bürkner, P., & Holling, H. (2018). Effects of expressive writing on depressive symptoms—A meta-analysis. *Clinical Psychology Science and Practice, 25*(1), e12224. https://doi.org/10.1111/cpsp.12224
29. Verduyn, P., Van Mechelen, I., Kross, E., Chezzi, C., & Van Bever, F. (2012). The relationship between self-distancing and the duration of negative and positive emotional experiences in daily life. *Emotion, 12*(6), 1248–1263. https://doi.org/10.1037/a0028289
30. Dorfman, A., Oakes, H., Santos, H. C., & Grossmann, I. (2019). Self-distancing promotes positive emotional change after adversity: Evidence from a micro-longitudinal field experiment. *Journal of Personality, 89*(1), 132–144. https://doi.org/10.1111/jopy.12534
31. Newman, K. M. (2016, November 9). Five science-backed strategies to build resilience. *Greater Good*. https://greatergood.berkeley.edu/article/item/five_science_backed_strategies_to_build_resilience

32. Burnett, D., Phillips, G., & Tashani, O. A. (2017). The effect of brief mindfulness meditation on cold-pressor induced pain responses in healthy adults. *Pain Studies and Treatment*, 5(2), 11–19. https://doi.org/10.4236/pst.2017.52002
33. Munroe, M., Al-Refae, M., Chan, H. W., & Ferrari, M. (2022). Using self-compassion to grow in the face of trauma: The role of positive reframing and problem-focused coping strategies. *Psychological Trauma Theory Research Practice and Policy*, 14(S1), S157–S164. https://doi.org/10.1037/tra0001164
34. Kyeong, S., Kim, J., Kim, D. J., Kim, H. E., & Kim, J. (2017). Effects of gratitude meditation on neural network functional connectivity and brain-heart coupling. *Scientific Reports*, 7(1). https://doi.org/10.1038/s41598-017-05520-9
35. Torre, J. B., & Lieberman, M. D. (2018). Putting feelings into words: Affect labeling as implicit emotion regulation. *Emotion Review*, 10(2), 116–124. https://doi.org/10.1177/1754073917742706
36. Kurland, B. (2024, March 25). Three ways to navigate difficult emotions. *Greater Good*. https://greatergood.berkeley.edu/article/item/three_ways_to_navigate_difficult_emotions
37. Kurland, B. (2019, January 14). What happens when you embrace dark emotions. *Greater Good*. https://greatergood.berkeley.edu/article/item/what_happens_when_you_embrace_dark_emotions
38. Bruehlman-Senecal, E., & Ayduk, O. (2015). This too shall pass: Temporal distance and the regulation of emotional distress. *Journal of Personality and Social Psychology*, 108(2), 356–375. https://doi.org/10.1037/a0038324
39. Newman, K. M. (2017, June 5). How comforting others helps you with your own struggles. *Greater Good*. https://greatergood.berkeley.edu/article/item/how_comforting_others_helps_you_with_your_own_struggles
40. Suttie, J. (2021, June 21). Does venting your feelings actually help? *Greater Good*. https://greatergood.berkeley.edu/article/item/does_venting_your_feelings_actually_help
41. Newman, K. M. (2021, February 8). How friends help you regulate your emotions. *Greater Good*. https://greatergood.berkeley.edu/article/item/how_friends_help_you_regulate_your_emotions
42. Newman, K. M. (2022, June 1). How your life is shaped by the emotions you want to feel. *Greater Good*. https://greatergood.berkeley.edu/article/item/how_your_life_is_shaped_by_the_emotions_you_want_to_feel
43. Hone, L. (2020, February 19). What I learned about resilience in the midst of grief. *Greater Good*. https://greatergood.berkeley.edu/article/item/what_i_learned_about_resilience_in_the_midst_of_grief

CHAPTER 10

1. Newman, K. M. (2020, July 14). How purpose changes across your lifetime. *Greater Good.* https://greatergood.berkeley.edu/article/item/how_purpose_changes_across_your_lifetime

2. Malin, H., Liauw, I., & Damon, W. (2017). Purpose and character development in early adolescence. *Journal of Youth and Adolescence, 46*(6), 1200–1215. https://doi.org/10.1007/s10964-017-0642-3

3. Ratner, K., Li, Q., Zhu, G., Estevez, M., & Burrow, A. L. (2023). Daily adolescent purposefulness, daily subjective well-being, and individual differences in autistic traits. *Journal of Happiness Studies, 24,* 957–989. https://doi.org/10.1007/s10902-023-00625-7

4. Barcaccia, B., Couyoumdjian, A., Di Consiglio, M., Papa, C., Cancellieri, U. G., & Cervin, M. (2023). Purpose in life as an asset for well-being and a protective factor against depression in adolescents. *Frontiers in Psychology, 14.* https://doi.org/10.3389/fpsyg.2023.1250279

5. Hill, P. L., Burrow, A. L., & Bronk, K. C. (2014). Persevering with positivity and purpose: An examination of purpose commitment and positive affect as predictors of grit. *Journal of Happiness Studies, 17*(1), 257–269. https://doi.org/10.1007/s10902-014-9593-5

6. Sharma, G., Kim, J., & Bernal-Arevalo, K. (2021). The relationship between high school sophomores' purpose orientations and their postsecondary completion a decade later. *Professional School Counseling, 25*(1). https://doi.org/10.1177/2156759x20981051

7. Hill, P. L., Burrow, A. L., Brandenberger, J. W., Lapsley, D. K., & Quaranto, J. C. (2010). Collegiate purpose orientations and well-being in early and middle adulthood. *Journal of Applied Developmental Psychology, 31*(2), 173–179. https://doi.org/10.1016/j.appdev.2009.12.001

8. Bronk, K. C., Hill, P. L., Lapsley, D. K., Talib, T. L., & Finch, H. (2009). Purpose, hope, and life satisfaction in three age groups. *The Journal of Positive Psychology, 4*(6), 500–510. https://doi.org/10.1080/17439760903271439

9. Sutin, A. R., Luchetti, M., Stephan, Y., Sesker, A. A., & Terracciano, A. (2024). Purpose in life and stress: An individual-participant meta-analysis of 16 samples. *Journal of Affective Disorders, 345,* 378–385. https://doi.org/10.1016/j.jad.2023.10.149

10. Boreham, I. D., & Schutte, N. S. (2023). The relationship between purpose in life and depression and anxiety: A meta-analysis. *Journal of Clinical Psychology, 79*(12), 2736–2767. https://doi.org/10.1002/jclp.23576

11. Bundick, M. J., Remington, K., Morton, E., & Colby, A. (2019). The contours of purpose beyond the self in midlife and later life. *Applied Developmental Science, 25*(1), 62–82. https://doi.org/10.1080/10888691.2018.1531718

12. Windsor, T. D., Curtis, R. G., & Luszcz, M. A. (2015). Sense of purpose as a psychological resource for aging well. *Developmental Psychology, 51*(7), 975–986. https://doi.org/10.1037/dev0000023

13. Steptoe, A., Deaton, A., & Stone, A. A. (2015). Subjective wellbeing, health, and ageing. *The Lancet, 385*(9968), 640–648. https://doi.org/10.1016/s0140-6736(13)61489-0
14. Sutin, A. R., Aschwanden, D., Luchetti, M., Stephan, Y., & Terracciano, A. (2021). Sense of purpose in life is associated with lower risk of incident dementia: A meta-analysis. *Journal of Alzheimer's Disease, 83*(1), 249–258. https://doi.org/10.3233/jad-210364
15. Kim, E. S., Sun, J. K., Park, N., Kubzansky, L. D., & Peterson, C. (2012). Purpose in life and reduced risk of myocardial infarction among older U.S. adults with coronary heart disease: A two-year follow-up. *Journal of Behavioral Medicine, 36*(2), 124–133. https://doi.org/10.1007/s10865-012-9406-4
16. Kim, E. S., Sun, J. K., Park, N., & Peterson, C. (2013). Purpose in life and reduced incidence of stroke in older adults: "The Health and Retirement Study." *Journal of Psychosomatic Research, 74*(5), 427–432. https://doi.org/10.1016/j.jpsychores.2013.01.013
17. Hill, P. L., & Turiano, N. A. (2014). Purpose in life as a predictor of mortality across adulthood. *Psychological Science, 25*(7), 1482–1486. https://doi.org/10.1177/0956797614531799
18. Turner, A. D., Smith, C. E., & Ong, J. C. (2017). Is purpose in life associated with less sleep disturbance in older adults? *Sleep Science and Practice, 1.* https://doi.org/10.1186/s41606-017-0015-6
19. Lewis, N. A., Turiano, N. A., Payne, B. R., & Hill, P. L. (2016). Purpose in life and cognitive functioning in adulthood. *Aging Neuropsychology and Cognition, 24*(6), 662–671. https://doi.org/10.1080/13825585.2016.1251549
20. Hill, P. L., Edmonds, G. W., & Hampson, S. E. (2017). A purposeful lifestyle is a healthful lifestyle: Linking sense of purpose to self-rated health through multiple health behaviors. *Journal of Health Psychology, 24*(10), 1392–1400. https://doi.org/10.1177/1359105317708251
21. Ma, X., Yang, Y., Lin, T., Zhang, Y., & Zheng, E. (2023). Loneliness, purpose in life, and protective behaviors: Examining cross-sectional and longitudinal relationships in older adults before and during COVID-19. *The Journals of Gerontology Series B, 78*(12), 2037–2044. https://doi.org/10.1093/geronb/gbad117
22. *Purpose in life quiz.* (2021, February). Greater Good. https://greatergood.berkeley.edu/quizzes/take_quiz/purpose_in_life
23. Schippers, M. C., Morisano, D., Locke, E. A., Scheepers, A. W., Latham, G. P., & De Jong, E. M. (2020). Writing about personal goals and plans regardless of goal type boosts academic performance. *Contemporary Educational Psychology, 60,* 101823. https://doi.org/10.1016/j.cedpsych.2019.101823
24. Wilson, K., & Groom, J. (2002). *Valued living questionnaire (VLQ).* Society of Clinical Psychology. Retrieved August 21, 2024, from https://www.div12.org/wp-content/uploads/2015/06/Valued-Living-Questionnaire.pdf
25. Schwartz, S. H. (2003). A proposal for measuring value orientations across nations. In *Questionnaire development package of the European social survey* (pp. 259–319). http://

www.europeansocialsurvey.org/docs/methodology/core_ess_questionnaire/ESS_core_questionnaire_human_values.pdf
26. Bronk, K. C., Baumsteiger, R., Mangan, S., Riches, B., Dubon, V., Benavides, C., & Bono, G. (2019). Fostering purpose among young adults: Effective online interventions. *Journal of Character Education, 15*(2), 21–38. https://eric.ed.gov/?id=EJ1232557
27. Bronk, K. C. (2011). A grounded theory of the development of noble youth purpose. *Journal of Adolescent Research, 27*(1), 78–109. https://doi.org/10.1177/0743558411412958
28. Damon, W. (2009). *The path to purpose: How young people find their calling in life*. Free Press.
29. *The 24 character strengths*. (n.d.). VIA Institute on Character. Retrieved August 22, 2024, from https://www.viacharacter.org/character-strengths
30. Smith, J. A. (2018, January 10). How to find your purpose in life. *Greater Good*. https://greatergood.berkeley.edu/article/item/how_to_find_your_purpose_in_life
31. Zakrzewski, V. (2018, April 12). How these teens found their sense of purpose. *Greater Good*. https://greatergood.berkeley.edu/article/item/how_these_teens_found_their_purpose_in_life
32. Suttie, J. (2015, May 12). How our bodies react to seeing goodness. *Greater Good*. https://greatergood.berkeley.edu/article/item/how_our_bodies_react_human_goodness
33. Han, H., Kim, J., Jeong, C., & Cohen, G. L. (2017). Attainable and relevant moral exemplars are more effective than extraordinary exemplars in promoting voluntary service engagement. *Frontiers in Psychology, 8*. https://doi.org/10.3389/fpsyg.2017.00283
34. Smith, J. A. (2018, January 10). How to find your purpose in life. *Greater Good*. https://greatergood.berkeley.edu/article/item/how_to_find_your_purpose_in_life
35. Newman, K. M. (2020, July 14). How purpose changes across your lifetime. *Greater Good*. https://greatergood.berkeley.edu/article/item/how_purpose_changes_across_your_lifetime
36. Hill, P. L., Sumner, R., & Burrow, A. L. (2014). Understanding the pathways to purpose: Examining personality and well-being correlates across adulthood. *The Journal of Positive Psychology, 9*(3), 227–234. https://doi.org/10.1080/17439760.2014.888584
37. *Beyond the self: 34 million older adults committed to common good*. (2018). CoGenerate. https://encore.org/wp-content/uploads/2018/03/PEP-Brief-2.pdf
38. Alboher, M. (2020, July 20). Find purpose by connecting across generations. *Greater Good*. https://greatergood.berkeley.edu/article/item/find_purpose_by_connecting_across_the_generations
39. Dhar, A. (2020, May 12). How I'm finding purpose and connection in a pandemic. *Greater Good*. https://greatergood.berkeley.edu/article/item/how_im_finding_purpose_and_connection_in_a_pandemic

CONCLUSION

1. Lyubomirsky, S. (2008). *The how of happiness: A new approach to getting the life you want.* Penguin Books.
2. Lyubomirsky, S. (n.d.). *Person-activity fit diagnostic.* The How of Happiness. https://thehowofhappiness.com/wp-content/themes/thehowofhappiness/Quiz/fit_diagnostic.html
3. De Witte, M. (2020, August 7). Is psychological research racially biased? *Greater Good.* https://greatergood.berkeley.edu/article/item/is_psychological_research_racially_biased
4. Tsai, J. L., Knutson, B., & Fung, H. H. (2006). Cultural variation in affect valuation. *Journal of Personality and Social Psychology, 90*(2), 288–307. https://doi.org/10.1037/0022-3514.90.2.288
5. Lyubomirsky, S., Sheldon, K. M., & Schkade, D. (2005). Pursuing happiness: The architecture of sustainable change. *Review of General Psychology, 9*(2), 111–131. https://doi.org/10.1037/1089-2680.9.2.111
6. Sheldon, K. M., Boehm, J. K., & Lyubomirsky, S. (2013). Variety is the spice of happiness: The hedonic adaptation prevention model. In S. A. David, I. Boniwell, & A. Conley Ayers (Eds.), *The Oxford handbook of happiness* (pp. 901–914). Oxford University Press. https://doi.org/10.1093/oxfordhb/9780199557257.013.0067
7. Carter, C. (2020, December 31). How to use immediate gratification to reach long-term goals. *Greater Good.* https://greatergood.berkeley.edu/article/item/how_to_use_immediate_gratification_to_reach_long_term_goals
8. Carter, C. (2014, December 30). The three most important tactics for keeping your resolutions. *Greater Good.* https://greatergood.berkeley.edu/article/item/the_three_most_important_tactics_for_keeping_your_resolutions
9. Newman, K. M. (2015, December 31). To change yourself, change your world. *Greater Good.* https://greatergood.berkeley.edu/article/item/to_change_yourself_change_your_world
10. Carter, C. (2017, August 29). How to get better at achieving your goals. *Greater Good.* https://greatergood.berkeley.edu/article/item/how_to_get_better_at_achieving_your_goals
11. Suttie, J. (2017, March 17). Which workplace policies help parents the most? *Greater Good.* https://greatergood.berkeley.edu/article/item/which_workplace_policies_help_parents_the_most
12. Smith, J. A. (2022, May 11). How much control do you have over your own happiness? *Greater Good.* https://greatergood.berkeley.edu/article/item/how_much_control_do_you_have_over_your_own_happiness
13. Newman, K. M. (2016, March 24). Why does happiness inequality matter? *Greater Good.* https://greatergood.berkeley.edu/article/item/why_does_happiness_inequality_matter
14. Newman, K. M. (2015, July 28). Six ways happiness is good for your health. *Greater Good.*

https://greatergood.berkeley.edu/article/item/six_ways_happiness_is_good_for_your_health

15. Fowler, J. H., & Christakis, N. A. (2008). Dynamic spread of happiness in a large social network: Longitudinal analysis over 20 years in the Framingham Heart Study. *BMJ, 337,* a2338. https://doi.org/10.1136/bmj.a2338

16. Suttie, J. (2019, September 11). Happiness doesn't make you ignore social problems. *Greater Good.* https://greatergood.berkeley.edu/article/item/happiness_doesnt_make_you_ignore_social_problems

17. Newman, K. M. (2014, December 22). Variety is the spice of emotional life. *Greater Good.* https://greatergood.berkeley.edu/article/item/variety_is_the_spice_of_emotional_life

18. Catalino, L. (2015, July 13). A better way to pursue happiness. *Greater Good.* https://greatergood.berkeley.edu/article/item/a_better_way_to_pursue_happiness

19. Mauss, I. B., Tamir, M., Anderson, C. L., & Savino, N. S. (2011). Can seeking happiness make people unhappy? Paradoxical effects of valuing happiness. *Emotion, 11*(4), 807–815. https://doi.org/10.1037/a0022010

20. Schooler, J. W., Ariel, Y. D., & Loewenstein, G. (2003). The pursuit and assessment of happiness can be self-defeating. In Isabelle Brocas & Juan D. Carrillo (Eds.), *The psychology of economic decisions: Rationality and well-being* (pp. 41–70). Oxford. https://doi.org/10.1093/oso/9780199251063.003.0003

21. Catalino, L. (2015, July 13). A better way to pursue happiness. *Greater Good.* https://greatergood.berkeley.edu/article/item/a_better_way_to_pursue_happiness

INDEX

abstinence
  gratitude and, 107
acceptance, 80, 82, 113, 117, 123, 132, 135, 160
Active Listening, 40–48
  in getting curious about others, 43
acts of kindness, 20–21
adaptive coping
  in emotion regulation, 128
ADHD. *see* attention-deficit hyperactivity disorder (ADHD)
affective empathy
  described, 35
Affect the Youth, 33
altruism, 20, 36
Amster, M., 78
anxious attachment
  described, 15
Armenta, C. N., 99
Arnold, A. B., 29
art design
  awe in, 76
attachment
  anxious, 15

avoidant, 15
disorganized, 15
secure, 4, 15
attachment styles
  described, 15
  reflection on, 16
  types of, 15–16
attention-deficit hyperactivity disorder (ADHD)
  case example, 111–12, 119
  Science of Happiness podcast on, 111–12
  self-compassion and, 111–12, 119
attitude(s)
  in emotion regulation, 134–35
avoidant attachment
  described, 15
awe, 64–79
  among Chinese people, 77
  behaviors/attitudes toward, 68–69
  benefits of, 65–68
  case example, 64–65, 79
  from children, 78
  described, 65
  experiencing of, 65–66

awe (*continued*)
   happiness related to, 67
   from inspirational person, 78
   life expectancy impact of, 68
   mental health impact of, 66–68
   from museum, 78
   negative, 68
   physical health impact of, 66–68
   practices related to, 70–75. *see also specific types and* awe practices
   quiz, 68–69
   relationships and, 65–66
   Science of Happiness podcast on, 64, 65
   specific experiences for, 75–77
   tips for cultivating, 77–79
   well-being impact of, 66–68
   your body and, 65–66
Awe Outing, 70–73
   described, 64–65, 79
awe practices, 70–75
   Awe Outing, 64–65, 70–73, 79
   Noticing Nature, 74–75
Awestruck, 78
Ayduk, O., 132

Barron, C., 22
Batson, C. D., 29
beauty
   awe in, 75
bias, 32, 38, 43–45, 84
Bilal, S., 140–41, 154–55
"Black Girl, Lost Keys," 119
body
   awe impact on, 65–66, 70–71, 77–78
   purpose impact on, 143–44
Body Scan meditation, 86–88
   described, 86–87

   Schneider on, 94–95
   Science of Happiness podcast on, 80–81
Boehm, J., 161–62
Brackett, M., 128
breathing
   mindful. *see* Mindful Breathing
bridging differences, 32, 38, 45, 77, 141, 154–155
bright side
   looking on, 137
Bronk, K. C., 149–51, 153
Brooks, R., 111, 119
Brown, B., 16
Buddhism, 52, 81
burnout, 37, 44, 53, 61

Camacho, B. R., 67
Cameron, C. D., 61
Capitalizing on Positive Events, 8–10
caregiver(s)
   forming secure attachment with, 4
Carter, J., 92
Catalino, L., 164
Celidwen, Y., 4
Center for Healthy Minds, 55–56
Center for Mindful Self-Compassion, 122–23
Cheavens, J., 30
children
   awe from, 78
Clarke, A., 108–9
closeness
   connection in achieving, 15–16
cognitive empathy
   described, 35
collective effervescence
   awe in, 76
Collins, H., 6
common ground

empathy in finding, 45–46
community(ies)
   in connection, 6–7
   of helpers, 62
compassion, 49–63
   behaviors/attitudes toward, 54–55
   benefits of, 51–54
   case example, 49–50, 62–63
   Dalai Lama on, 52
   described, 51, 59
   empathy vs., 50–51
   happiness related to, 52–53
   health related to, 53–54
   kindness vs., 50–51
   methods of, 59–61
   practices related to, 55–59, 62–63. *see also specific types and* compassion practices
   relationships impact of, 51–52
   self-, 111–24. *see also* self-compassion
   specific indications for, 59–63
   trauma victims impact from, 53
   Tutu on, 52
   well-being impact of, 51
compassion fatigue
   avoiding, 61–63
Compassion Meditation, 55–57, 62–63
   reflection on, 57
   Science of Happiness podcast on, 62–63
compassion practices, 55–59, 62–63
   Compassion Meditation, 55–57, 62–63
   Feeling Supported, 57–59
connected
   feeling, 10–11
connected communities, 6–7
connection, 1–17
   behaviors/attitudes toward, 7
   benefits of, 2–3
   case example, 1–2, 8, 14, 17
   communities in, 6–7
   feelings of, 7–8
   happiness related to, 3, 6–7, 97
   importance of, 3–4, 98
   in getting closer, 15–16
   levels of, 14–15
   loneliness and, 1–2, 13–15
   nurturing of, 3
   opening up in, 16–17
   practices related to, 8–13. *see also specific types and* connection practices
   reflections on, 6, 7
   relationships in, 5–6. *see also* relationship(s)
   roots of, 4–7
   Science of Happiness podcast on, 8
   social. *see* social connections
   specific indications for, 13–17
   with strangers, 5–6
connection practices, 8–13
   Capitalizing on Positive Events, 8–10
   Feeling Connected, 10–11
   Small Talk, 6, 11–13
connective moments
   types of, 17
conversation(s)
   with friends, 15
coping
   adaptive. *see* adaptive coping
COVID-19 pandemic
   gratitude impact on, 98
culture
   in Happiness Plan, 157–58
curiosity
   about others, 43

Dalai Lama
　on compassion, 52
Damon, W., 151
Darley, J. M., 29
death
　awe in encountering, 77
Depow, G., 38
Desmond, T., 122
DeSteno, D., 37
difficult times
　gratitude during, 108–9
disorganized attachment
　described, 15
distancing
　self-. *see* self-distancing

Eagle, J., 78
effervescence
　awe in, 76
Emmons, R. A., 97, 98, 108–9
emotion(s)
　positive. *see* positive emotions
　regulation of. *see* emotion regulation
　social. *see* social emotion
　unpleasant. *see* unpleasant emotions
emotional intelligence
　in emotion regulation, 128
emotion regulation, 125–39
　adaptive coping in, 128
　behaviors/attitudes toward, 129
　benefits of, 128
　case example, 125–26, 138–39
　cultivating forgiveness in, 136–37
　described, 126
　emotional intelligence in, 128
　healthy, 128
　imaging future in, 135
　looking on bright side in, 137
　naming your feelings in, 134

　practices for, 130–34. *see also specific types and* emotion regulation practices
　seeing what you can learn in, 135
　seeking positive emotions in, 137–39
　sharing your troubles with others in, 136
　soothing practices in, 135
　specific indications for, 134–39
　taking open/welcoming/accepting attitude in, 134–35
　value of unpleasant emotions in, 137
　working with unpleasant emotions in, 126–28. *see also under* unpleasant emotions
emotion regulation practices, 130–34
　Expressive Writing, 125–26, 130–32
　Gaining Perspective on Negative Events, 132–35
emotion suppression
　described, 127–28
empathic distress, 44–45
empathy, 34–48
　across our differences, 37–39
　affective, 35
　in avoiding distress/overwhelm, 44–45
　behaviors/attitudes toward, 39–40
　benefits of, 35–39
　case example, 34–35, 47–48
　cognitive, 35
　compassion vs., 50–51
　described, 35, 38
　elements of, 35–36
　in finding common ground, 45–46
　in getting curious about others, 43
　happiness related to, 36–37
　in helping others, 36
　offering of, 35
　positive feelings–related, 38
　practices related to, 40–48. *see also specific types and* empathy practices

quiz, 39–40
   receiving of, 35
   in romantic relationships, 37
   specific indications for, 43–46, 48
   in work environment, 37
empathy practices, 40–48
   Active Listening, 40–48
   Shared Identity, 46–47
environment(s)
   in mindfulness, 83
Epel, E., 127
epiphanies
   awe in, 77
esteem
   self-. see self-esteem
Eva, A. L., 44–45
exercise, 14, 135
expressing thanks
   gratitude and, 107
Expressive Writing, 125–26, 130–32
   Science of Happiness podcast on, 125–26

family(ies)
children, 20, 36, 78, 99
parents, 14, 51, 151
relatives, 22, 141
   relationships outside of, 5
Farm to Family, 153
fatigue
   compassion. see compassion fatigue
feeling(s)
   of connectedness, 7–8
   of loneliness, 1–2
   naming of, 134
   positive. see positive feelings
Feeling Connected, 10–11
Feeling Supported, 57–59
fierce self-compassion
   components of, 123–24

Fierce Self-Compassion Break reflection
   Neff's, 124
finding purpose
   patience in, 154–55
   reflecting on yourself/your life/the world in, 151–53
   trying out new things in, 153–54
focus on others
   gratitude and, 108
forgiveness
   cultivating, 136–37
friend(s)
conversations with, 15, 136–137, 152
friendship(s)
   happiness related to, 3–5, 14–15
   Science of Happiness course on, 5
future
   imagining of, 135

Gable, S., 8
Gaining Perspective on Negative Events, 132–35
Gameros, D., xviii, 64–65, 79
generosity, 20, 55
Germer, C., 122, 124
getting closer
   connection in, 15–16
GGSC. see Greater Good Science Center (GGSC)
Gift of Time, 26–27
good
   taking in of, 107
Grander, T., 28
gratitude, 96–110
   abstinence and, 107
   behaviors/attitudes toward, 100–1
   benefits of, 97–99
   case example, 96–97, 103–4
   COVID-19 pandemic impact of, 98

gratitude (continued)
    described, 106
    in embracing our interdependence, 109–10
    expressing, 98–99
    expressing thanks and, 107
    focusing on others and, 108
    going through the motions in, 108
    in hard times, 108–9
    imagination and, 106–7
    for mental health, 97–98
    for physical health, 97–98
    practices for, 101–6. *see also specific types and* gratitude practices
    quiz, 100–101
    relationships impact of, 98–99
    repeated practice of, 108
    savoring and, 107
    as social emotion, 98
    specific indications for, 106–8
    taking in the good and, 107
    well-being impact of, 97–98
Gratitude Journal, 101–3
    benefits from, 97, 101
    guidelines for keeping, 101–3
Gratitude Letter, 96–97, 103–6
    Science of Happiness podcast on, 96–97
gratitude practices, 101–6
    Gratitude Journal, 101–3
    Gratitude Letter, 103–6
Gray, H., 49, 80, 111
Greater Good in Action website, xv–xvi
Greater Good magazine, xiv–xv
Greater Good Science Center (GGSC), xix–xx
    described, xiv
    on happiness, 163
    Purpose Challenge Scholarship Contest of, 152

habits, xvii, 92, 144, 157
Hanson, R., 60, 62, 107
happiness
    acknowledging what you can't control in, 162–63
    awe impact on, 67
    causes of, xiii
    compassion impact on, 52–53
    described, xvi–xvii
    don't obsess over, 163–64
    empathy impact on, 36–37
    friendships related to, 5
    keys to, xvii–xviii
    kindness impact on, 20–21
    moments of, xiii–xiv
    nurturing of social connections in, 3
    plan for, 157–64. *see also* Happiness Plan
    reflection on, 158–59
    relationships and, 5–6
    variety and, 161–62
    well-being and, xvi–xvii
Happiness Plan, 157–64
    acknowledging what you can't control in, 162–63
    components of, 159–60
    cultural background in, 157–58
    don't obsess over happiness in, 163–64
    obstacles in, 161
    practices in, 157–62
    variety in, 161–62
Harvard's School of Public Health, 143–44
Harvey, A., xviii, 18–20, 29, 33
health
    compassion impact on, 37, 53–54
    kindness impact on, 22
    mental. *see* mental health
    physical. *see* physical health
helper(s)
    community of, 62

helping others
  empathy in, 36
  when you need help, 30–31
Higginsen, "Mama" Vy, 154
Hill, P. L., 144
Holmes, C. M., 29–30
Hone, L., 137–38
hormone(s)
oxytocin, 51, 66
Hougaard, R., 92
How Would You Treat A Friend?, 119–21
Hunt, C., 92
Hunt, L., 76

idea(s)
  awe in, 77
identity(ies)
  shared. *see* Shared Identity
illness(es)
  loneliness-related, 2
imagination
  gratitude and, 106–7
informal mindfulness, 92–95
inspirational person
  awe from, 78
intelligence
  emotional. *see* emotional intelligence
interdependence
  gratitude in embracing, 109–10
In the Form of a Question: The Rewards and Joys of a Curious Life, 95

Jasir, T., 5
Jazaieri, H., 61, 91–92, 94
John, K., 60
Jordan, M., 152
journal(s)
  gratitude, 97, 101–3. *see also* Gratitude Journal

Kabat-Zinn, J., 81, 92, 93
Kabul Dreams, 125–26, 139
Kalantari, S.
  background of, xiv–xv
  on *Science of Happiness* podcast, xv, xviii
Karg, K., 76
Kashdan, T., 109–10
Keltner, D., 59, 68
Kim, E. S., 143–44
kind acts, 20–21
kindness, 18–33
  acts of, 20–21
  awkwardness of, 28–29
  barriers to, 31
  behaviors/attitudes toward, 23–24
  benefits of, 20–23
  case example, 18–20, 29, 33
  challenges-related reflection, 31
  compassion vs., 50–51
  as contagious, 22–23
  examples of, 20
  expanding one's, 31–33
  finding shared identity in, 32
  finding what motivates you in, 32–33
  happiness related to, 20–21
  health effects of, 22
  helping others when you need help, 30–31
  impacts of, 20–23, 28–29
  life of, 33
  observing impact of, 32
  practices related to, 24–27. *see also specific types and* kindness practices
  quiz, 23–24
  reflection on, 21
  relationships effects of, 22–23
  self-, 31
  specific indications for, 28–33
  spending money related to, 21

kindness (*continued*)
    time and energy for, 29–30
    toward others, 15
kindness practices, 24–27
    awkwardness-related, 28–29
    Gift of Time, 26–27
    Random Acts of Kindness, 24–26
King, M. L., Jr., 18
Klimecki, O., 52–53
Koerber, K., 96–97, 103–4
Krznaric, R., 43
Kurland, B., 127, 134–35

Laurent, S., 66
letter(s)
    gratitude, 96–97, 103–6. see also Gratitude Letter
Levasseur, A., 71
Lieberman, M. D., 4
life
    awe in encountering, 77
    reflecting on, 151–53
Life Crafting, 146–49
    defined, 146
life expectancy
    awe impact on, 68
life of kindness, 33
Light, W., 30
Lindsay, E., 82
listening
    active, 40–48. see also Active Listening
listening skills
    Science of Happiness podcast on, 48
loneliness
    antidotes to, 14
    as common struggle, 14
    connection and, 1–2, 13–15
    coping skills for, 14–15
    described, 2
    feelings of, 1–2
    illnesses related to, 2
    Office of the Surgeon General on, 1–2
    stigma related to, 14
longevity
    well-being and, 2–3
Lyubomirsky, S., 20, 22, 99, 157, 161–62

Magic Wand, 140–41, 149–50, 154–55
Mailbom, H., 43
Malcolm X, 18
Mama Foundation for the Arts, 154
Marjory Stoneman Douglas High School Parkland, FL, 96–97
Max Planck Institute, 52–53
Maxworthy, G., 153
MBSR. *see* Mindfulness-Based Stress Reduction (MBSR)
meaning, xiv, 5, 20, 71, 137
meditation(s)
    Body Scan. *see* Body Scan meditation
    Metta, 52
    Mindful Breathing, 88–91
Mehta, N., 27
mental health
    awe impact on, 66–68
    gratitude for, 97–98
    self-compassion impact on, 112–115
Metta meditation, 52
Mindful Breathing, 88–91
    described, 88–90
mindfulness, 80–95
    in action, 93
    behaviors/attitudes toward, 84–85
    benefits of, 81–84
    described, 81
    environments in, 83
    informal, 92–95
    for performance, 82–83

practices of, 86–91. *see also specific types and* mindfulness practices
quiz, 84–85
relationships impact of, 83–84
Science of Happiness course on, 94
specific indications for, 91–95
for stress, 81–82
tips for incorporating, 93–94
for well-being, 82–83
Mindfulness-Based Stress Reduction (MBSR), 81
mindfulness in action, 93
mindfulness practices, 86–91
Body Scan meditation, 80–81, 86–88, 94–95
Mindful Breathing, 88–91
types of, 83
Mindful Self-Compassion program, 122
mirror neurons, 35
money
kindness and, 21
moral beauty
awe in, 75
moral elevation, 23
Morgan-Jones, J., 66
motivation
kindness and, 32–33
Murthy, V., xviii, 1–2, 8, 14, 17
museum
awe from, 78
music
awe in, 76

naming of feelings, 134
nature
awe in, 76
Neff, K., 112, 114, 116, 119–24
Fierce Self-Compassion Break reflection of, 124
negative awe, 68

negative events
gaining perspective on, 132–35
neuron(s)
mirror, 35
Newman, K. M.
background of, xiv
Noticing Nature, 74–75
nurturing
of social connections, 3

Office of the Surgeon General
on loneliness, 1–2
Ontiveros, E., 34–35, 47–48
opening up
in connection, 16–17
others
curiosity about, 43
focusing on, 108
helping of. *see* helping others
kindness toward, 15
sharing your troubles with, 136
overwhelm
empathy in avoiding, 44–45
oxytocin
as tend and befriend hormone, 66
well-being effects of, 51

Papaioannou, Y., 94
Paquette, J., 78
Passmore, H.-A., 74–75
patience
in finding purpose, 154–55
Pennebaker, J. W., 130
performance
mindfulness for, 82–83
physical health
awe impact of, 66–68
compassion impact on, 53–54
gratitude for, 97–98

positive emotions
  seeking of, 137–39
positive feelings
  empathy related to, 38
positive psychology
  described, xiv–xv
psychological richness
  described, xvi
psychology
  positive, xiv–xv
purpose, 140–55
  behaviors/attitudes toward, 144–45
  benefits of, 142–44
  case example, 140–41, 154–55
  good for mind/good for body, 143–44
  practices for, 146–50. *see also specific types and* purpose practices
  quiz, 144–145
  Science of Happiness podcast on, 140–41
  sense of. *see* sense of purpose
  specific ways for finding, 150–55. *see also under* finding purpose
  well-being impact of, 142–43
Purpose Challenge Scholarship Contest of GGSC, 152
purpose practices, 146–50
  Life Crafting, 146–49
  Magic Wand, 140–41, 149–50

Qardash, S., 125–26, 138–39

racism, 112, 162
Raj, Rexx Life, 49–50, 62–63
Random Acts of Kindness, 24–26
  Science of Happiness podcast on, 18–19
reflection
  on attachment styles, 16
  on Compassion Meditation, 57
  on connection, 6, 7
  Fierce Self-Compassion Break, 124
  on happiness, 158–59
  kindness-related, 21
  kindness-related challenges, 31
  on trust, 16
  on vulnerability, 16
  on yourself/your life/the world, 151–53
regulation
  emotion, 125–39. *see also* emotion regulation
relationship(s)
  awe impact on, 65–66
  compassion impact on, 51–52
  empathy in, 37
  gratitude impact on, 98–99
  happiness related to, 5–6
  kindness impact on, 22–23
  mindfulness impact on, 83–84
  outside of immediate families, 5
  self-compassion impact on, 114
  types of, 5–6
  well-being impact of, 3
religion
  awe in, 76
Ren, D., 14
resilience
  self-compassion and, 53, 81–82, 113–14, 128
Riess, H., 36
romantic relationships
  empathy in, 37
RULER, 128
Rumi, 44

Sahi, R., 136
Sankararaman, A., 117
savoring

gratitude and, 107
Schneider, A., 80–81
   on Body Scan meditation, 94–95
Science of Happiness course, xix
   on friendships, 5
   mindfulness in, 94
Science of Happiness podcast, xx
   on ADHD, 111–12
   on awe, 64, 65
   on Body Scan meditation, 80–81
   on Compassion Meditation, 62–63
   on connection, 8
   on Expressive Writing, 125–26
   on Gratitude Letter, 96–97
   Kalantari on, xv, xviii
   on listening skills, 48
   on purpose, 140–41
   on Random Acts of Kindness, 18–19
secure attachment
   described, 15
   forming, 4
self
   reflecting on, 151–53
self-compassion, 111–24
   ADHD and, 111–12, 119
   behaviors/attitudes toward, 115–16
   benefits of, 112–14
   case example, 111–12, 119
   Center for Mindful Self-Compassion on, 122–23
   components of, 112
   fierce, 123–24
   in improving one's life, 113–14
   mental health impact of, 113
   quiz, 115–116
   practices for, 116–21. *see also specific types and* self-compassion practices

relationships impact from, 114
   resilience and, 113–14
   resistance to, 114–15
   self-esteem vs., 113
   specific indications for, 121–24
   tender, 123
Self-Compassionate Letter, 116–19
   case example, 111–12, 119
self-compassion practices, 116–21
   How Would You Treat A Friend?, 119–21
   Self-Compassionate Letter, 111–12, 116–19
self-distancing
   described, 132–34
   practice for, 132–34
self-esteem
   self-compassion vs., 113
self-kindness, 31
Seligman, M., xv
sense(s)
   appreciation of, 78
sense of purpose, 140–55. *see also under* purpose
   COVID-19 pandemic impact on, 144
   described, 142–43
ServiceSpace, 27
Shared Identity, 46–47
   kindness and, 32
Sheldon, K. M., 161–62
Sheridan, L., 77–78
Shin, J., 60
sleep, 14, 67, 144
Simon-Thomas, E., 44
Small Talk, 6, 11–13
Smith, J. A., 153, 163
Social: Why Our Brains Are Wired to Connect, 4

social emotion
   gratitude as, 98
social ties
   importance of, 5
   looser, 5
Societal Reform Corporation, 96
soothing practices
   in emotion regulation, 135
spirituality
   awe in, 76
Stanford Center on Adolescence, 151
Stavrova, O., 14
strangers
   connection with, 5–6
stress
   mindfulness for, 81–82
"subjective" well-being, xvi
suffering
   unmasking/masking of, 60
suppression
   of emotions, 127–28
Suttie, J.
   background of, xiv–xv
Svoboda, E., 59–60, 62

taking in the good
   gratitude and, 107
talk
   small. see Small Talk
technology
   unplug from, 78
tend-and-befriend hormone
   oxytocin as, 66
tender self-compassion
   components of, 123
thanks
   expressing, 107
The Blue Hour, 49–50

The Empathy Effect, 36
The How of Happiness, 22, 157
"The Power of Vulnerability," 16
The Stress Prescription, 127
Thnx4.org, 107
Together: The Healing Power of Human Connection in a Sometimes Lonely World, 17
trauma
   compassion impact on, 53
   PTSD, 34, 47, 53, 67, 113
   victims of. see victims of trauma
trust
   reflection on, 16
trying out new things
   in finding purpose, 153–54
Tutu, D., 52

UCLA Mindful, 86, 89
unhappiness
   recipe for, xvii
unpleasant emotions
   benefits of working with, 126–28
   reminding yourself of value of, 137
unplug from technology, 78

variety
   happiness and, 161–62
victims of trauma
   compassion in helping, 53
visual design
   awe in, 76
vulnerability
   embracing, 16
   reflection on, 16

Watelet, C., 94
Weiss, L., 92–93
well-being

awe impact on, 66–68
compassion impact on, 51
described, xvi–xvii
gratitude impact on, 97–98
happiness and, xvi–xvii
longevity related to, 2–3
mindfulness for, 82–83
oxytocin impact on, 51
relationships in, 3
sense of purpose impact on, 142–43
"subjective," xvi
Weng, H., 55–56
work environment
    empathy in, 37
world
    reflection on, 151–53
writing
    expressive. *see* Expressive Writing

ABOUT THE AUTHORS

Based at the University of California, Berkeley, the **Greater Good Science Center** studies the psychology, sociology, and neuroscience of well-being, and teaches skills that foster a thriving, resilient, and compassionate society. Its programs include *Greater Good* magazine and *The Science of Happiness* podcast.

Kira M. Newman is the managing editor of *Greater Good* magazine at UC Berkeley's Greater Good Science Center. Her work has been published in a variety of outlets, including *The Washington Post*, *HuffPost*, *Mindful* magazine, and TED Ideas, and she is coeditor of *The Gratitude Project* (New Harbinger, 2020). She has created large communities around the science of happiness, including the online course The Year of Happy as well as the CaféHappy meetup in Toronto, Canada. Kira is also a personal trainer at New Element Training and was previously a technology journalist and editor for *Tech.Co*.

Jill Suttie, PsyD, is a former practicing psychologist turned freelance science journalist. For the past 20 years, she's been a writer at *Greater Good* magazine, covering research on compassion, forgiveness, mindfulness, purpose, awe, humility, nature experiences, and more. Through articles and book reviews, she translates scientific findings and provides useful tips for personal and societal well-being. Outside of *Greater Good*, her writing has appeared in *Huff Post*, *The Washington Post*, *Mindful*, and *Yes! Magazine*, among others, and she's been a featured podcast speaker. In her free time, she enjoys traveling, hiking, socializing, singing, and playing guitar.

Shuka Kalantari is the executive producer of audio for the award-winning podcast, *The Science of Happiness*. Her background is in healthcare journalism and narrative story-telling, focusing on the intersection between health, community, and social justice. Her work has appeared on *The World* by PRX, BBC World News Service's *Outlook*, KQED public radio, and in *VICE*, among others.